Mobilizing Against AIDS

Mobilizing Against AIDS

The Unfinished Story of a Virus

Institute of Medicine
National Academy of Sciences
Eve K. Nichols, Writer

HARVARD UNIVERSITY PRESS
Cambridge, Massachusetts
London, England
1986

This book is printed on acid-free paper, and its binding materials have been chosen for strength and durability.

Library of Congress Cataloging in Publication Data

Mobilizing Against AIDS.

   Drawn from the 1985 Annual Meeting of the Institute
of Medicine.
   Bibliography: p.
   Includes index.
   1. AIDS (Disease)—Congresses. I. Institute of
Medicine (U.S.). Meeting (1985: Washington, D.C.)
[DNLM: 1. Acquired Immunodeficiency Syndrome.
2. Health Policy. WD 308 M687]
RC607.A26M63   1986   616.9'792   86-80832

ISBN 0-674-57760-4
ISBN 0-674-57761-2 (pbk.)

To Frederick C. Robbins, M.D., immediate past president of the Institute of Medicine, whose pioneering work earlier in this century helped to eliminate the fearsome viral disease polio

Preface

Few diseases in modern times have raised such fears and uncertainties as the acquired immune deficiency syndrome (AIDS) and the malignancies, infections, and brain damage that can accompany it. In little more than five years AIDS has grown from a clinical oddity to a virtual epidemic, half of whose victims already have died and the vast majority of whom will be dead within three years of their seeking medical attention. At the same time, stunning successes in the sciences of molecular biology and epidemiology have led to discovery and description in intricate detail of the virus that causes AIDS and the major pathways of its spread. But medical science has not yet been able to create a vaccine against the virus or a drug that can prevent or quell infection by it.

Already, thousands of cases of AIDS in the United States are beginning to strain the capacity and deplete the resources of hospitals, physicians, nurses, and others in the cities hardest hit by the disease. A constantly increasing population of AIDS patients will severely burden the health care system, including the components of science and education that underpin it.

The spreading peril of AIDS prompted the Institute of Medicine to devote the scientific session of its 1985 annual meeting to a wide-ranging examination of the disease, from its devastation of the human body to its disruption of society. This book is drawn from that meeting. It reports the triumphs in the newest laboratory investigations of AIDS, the clinical complexities of the disease, the possibilities for prevention and treatment, and the ethical and psychosocial difficulties posed by the disease. In addition, appendixes provide U.S. Public Health Service recommendations for preventing infection in the workplace, for reducing the risks of transmitting AIDS, and for the care of infected children.

The presentations underscore the need for public policy decisions that can establish funding for the care of AIDS victims, identify and apportion responsibilities for needed scientific research, and foster the programs for education and behavioral change that currently are the primary means of controlling the disease.

The specific views in the book are a composite of ideas presented by the speakers, whose contributions are acknowledged at the end of each chapter, and do not represent the full range of contemporary opinions on public policy and ethical issues. The ideas and conclusions expressed at the meeting, however, have contributed to the convening of a larger body of scientists, health care practitioners, public health leaders, and others to study how the nation's responses to AIDS can be brought to maximum effectiveness.

Samuel O. Thier
President, Institute of Medicine

April 1986

Contents

1. The Scope of AIDS   1

2. Tracking the Epidemic   10

3. The Spectrum of Disease   41

4. Discovery of the Virus   59

5. Damage to the Immune System and the Brain   74

6. Prevention and Treatment   89

7. Individual and Societal Stress   118

8. Public Health Policy   132

Appendixes

A. Current CDC Definition of AIDS   149

B. PHS Recommendations for Preventing Transmission of Infection with HTLV-III/LAV in the Workplace   155

C.   Additional PHS Recommendations to Reduce
Sexual and Drug Abuse–Related Transmission
of HTLV–III/LAV   172

D.   PHS Recommendations: Education and Foster
Care of Children Infected with HTLV–III/LAV   178

E.   Organizations to Contact for Information
on AIDS   185

Suggested Readings   189

Glossary   191

Contributors and Acknowledgments   197

Index   199

Mobilizing Against AIDS

1

The Scope of AIDS

He put his cane down on the table next to his bed and slowly removed his shirt. The sunlight streaming through the window fell on his chest as he turned reluctantly toward the mirror. For weeks he had been afraid to look at his own reflection. The purplish spots of Kaposi's sarcoma now covered his entire torso. The boyish face crumpled and he cried as he had many times during the past eighteen months. He was twenty-four years old and he knew that the infections raging through his body would kill him before the spring.

The American public has read hundreds of such accounts describing lonely battles against one of the most publicized killers of this century, acquired immune deficiency syndrome (AIDS). AIDS cripples the body's defense mechanisms, leaving them unable to fight even the least aggressive bacteria and other microorganisms. It is caused by the virus HTLV-III/LAV (human T-cell lymphotropic virus type III/lymphadenopathy-associated virus). Public health experts believe that a million or more Americans have already been infected with HTLV-III/LAV.

No one knows how many of those infected will eventually become sick. Among infected homosexual men enrolled in a long-term study in San Francisco, 6.4 percent developed AIDS within five years. (Less serious AIDS-related conditions were identified in 25.8 percent.) Among other groups of infected persons the reported AIDS incidence rates have been substantially higher—ranging from 8.0 to 34.2 percent over

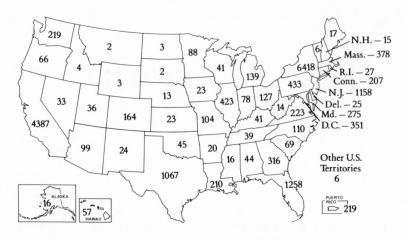

FIGURE 1. AIDS cases (total = 19,181) reported to the Centers for Disease Control by each of the 50 states, the District of Columbia, and three U.S. territories through April 4, 1986. Source: U.S. Department of Health and Human Services, Public Health Service, Centers for Disease Control.

three years in five study groups followed by the National Cancer Institute's James J. Goedert and his colleagues.

The Centers for Disease Control (CDC) in Atlanta has received notification of AIDS cases from all 50 states, the District of Columbia, and three U.S. territories (see Figure 1). As of April 1986, more than 19,000 AIDS cases had been reported; more than 10,000 of the patients had died. Experts expect that a total of 14,000 to 15,000 new cases of AIDS will be diagnosed in 1986 and that at least 7,000 AIDS patients will die.

The long lag time between initial infection and the appearance of disease—up to five years or more—complicates efforts to make long-term predictions about the course of the epidemic. The rate of increase in the number of cases appears to be slowing down gradually. In 1983 the number of cases was doubling about every 6 months; the most recent doubling took 11 months, and public health experts predict that the next doubling will take about 13 months. Nonetheless, the absolute number of cases continues to rise sharply.

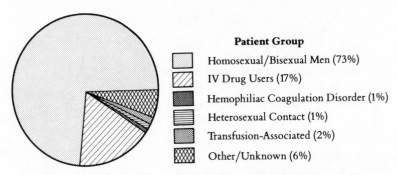

FIGURE 2.   Reported adult cases of AIDS (total = 18,907) in the United States: percentage by patient group, 1981 to April 4, 1986. (Eleven percent of the homosexual/bisexual males reported having used intravenous [IV] drugs.) Source: U.S. Department of Health and Human Services, Public Health Service, Centers for Disease Control.

Those most familiar with the devastating effects of the syndrome are the nation's homosexuals (see Figure 2). AIDS continues to occur primarily among homosexuals, intravenous drug abusers and their sexual partners, and individuals who received blood or blood products before techniques were developed to safeguard the blood supply. The proportion of cases occurring outside these high-risk groups has remained small and constant, at about 6 percent.

In cities across the United States, homosexuals describe the anguish of watching one friend after another weaken and die. The loss of a dozen friends in less than six months is not uncommon in cities hardest hit by the epidemic: New York City, San Francisco, Los Angeles, Miami, Washington, D.C., and Houston. Most of the dead have been young men (more than 90 percent of AIDS patients are between the ages of 20 and 49). June E. Osborn, dean of the School of Public Health at the University of Michigan, describes the loss in human terms: "We are losing a generation of well-trained and exceptionally talented men, and humanity cannot afford to lose even an iota of trained talent in these troubled times."

The economic impact is equally grave. CDC scientists have calculated the loss in productivity resulting from the disability and premature deaths of the first 10,000 AIDS patients. That loss alone, they estimate, will total more than $4.8 billion. This figure does not include productivity losses stemming from other problems related to HTLV-III/LAV infection. Among these are the clinical and immunological abnormalities covered under the term AIDS-related complex (ARC), and the mental and physical handicaps caused by viral invasion of the nervous system in persons whose immune systems may appear normal.

The wide range of potential consequences of infection with HTLV-III/LAV (see Chapter 3) makes it very difficult to assess the ultimate impact of this epidemic. Almost two-thirds of infected men participating in the long-term CDC study in San Francisco have remained healthy for more than five years, but scientists fear that at least some will develop HTLV-III/LAV-related illnesses as they grow older.

Researchers in laboratories across the country have begun searching for clues that will explain why some individuals are more susceptible than others to AIDS and related conditions. These studies, like most other aspects of AIDS research, would not have been possible without recently developed techniques in molecular biology, virology, and recombinant DNA technology. Says Dr. Osborn:

> I have often mused about how we would be coping now if we lacked viral culture and cell sorting techniques, detailed knowledge about the replication of retroviruses, and monoclonal antibodies, to name just a few of the advances that appeared to be highly esoteric when they were first introduced into the biomedical sciences. Without them, we would have had difficulty phrasing even the most elementary questions about what was happening to the thousands of young persons plagued by almost-unheard-of microbes and tumors.

The pace of AIDS research has been extraordinary. Scientists in France and the United States isolated and identified HTLV-III/LAV less than three years after AIDS was first described by physicians in California and New York. Less than a year later, researchers had developed a rapid screening test to limit the spread of infection through blood products and to identify those at greatest risk of disease.

Early attempts to assess the effects of HTLV-III/LAV on human defense mechanisms resulted in an apparent paradox: although the broad range of clinical signs and symptoms associated with AIDS suggested multiple problems crippling many different aspects of the immune response, a closer look showed a much more specific defect. The virus was incapacitating a very special type of white blood cell—a cell that coordinates the activities of other immune cells. Without this "helper" cell, the body cannot respond effectively to many external challenges.

Unfortunately, the more scientists have learned about HTLV-III/LAV the less sanguine they have become about the prospects for rapid solutions to the AIDS problem. Several characteristics of the virus make it an extremely tough opponent. Its genetic information rapidly integrates itself into the genetic machinery of human target cells. The only way to eradicate it is to kill the infected cells. This appeared feasible when scientists believed that the virus infected only certain populations of white blood cells—the body can be induced to replace blood cells—but new evidence indicates that HTLV-III/LAV also has a predilection for brain cells. Scientists do not yet know whether the brain cells that harbor the virus are irreplaceable nerve cells or other components of neural tissues.

AIDS probably is not a curable disease, but it may be treatable. If scientists can inhibit replication of the virus, they may be able to prevent it from spreading from one cell to another inside the body. This might be sufficient to control clinical symptoms: patients would live normal lives as long as they continued to take an appropriate antiviral drug.

Several different kinds of drugs have been shown to suppress replication of HTLV-III/LAV in the test tube, but none has produced long-term clinical improvement in AIDS patients. Scientists at the National Institutes of Health are overseeing drug trials at selected U.S. medical centers. No one can predict, however, when a suitable drug or drug combination will be ready for widespread use.

The possibility of an AIDS vaccine is even less certain than that of developing an antiviral drug. In early 1984, Margaret M. Heckler, then secretary of the U.S. Department of Health and Human Services, predicted that a vaccine might be ready for clinical trials in two years. Seventeen months later, a long-range plan to control AIDS developed by the Public Health Service acknowledged that it was unlikely that a vaccine would be generally available before 1990.

At least one vaccine candidate is undergoing tests in laboratory animals, but even if it passes these tests, the road to a human vaccine will be long and arduous. The logistics and expense of clinical trials present enormous barriers to vaccine development, and there are many questions about who would make such a vaccine and who should receive it.

For now, the only way to slow the spread of AIDS is through education and other public health measures. The types of behavior most likely to transmit the virus are well known: sexual contact with a member of a high-risk group and the sharing of intravenous needles and syringes by drug abusers. Women who are infected can transmit the virus to their unborn and newborn babies. Studies of thousands of health care workers and the families of AIDS victims have found no evidence that the disease can be transmitted by casual contact.

Persuading individuals to change long-term habits of sexual behavior or drug abuse is extremely difficult, but recent evidence indicates that carefully designed programs can be effective. It is equally important to ensure that adolescents understand the risk of AIDS. For many teenagers in the United States, experimentation extends to sexual experiences and the use of intravenous drugs. Information on AIDS should be included in existing programs to discourage indiscriminate sex and drug abuse.

Policymakers in geographic areas that have not been severely affected by the AIDS crisis should not wait to implement these programs until the situation becomes worse. As indicated above, the long latency period and the large number of infected persons without symptoms make it very difficult to assess the dimensions of the problem. To be most effective, prevention efforts must get under way before the virus becomes prevalent in a community.

Widespread education also will help allay the fears about AIDS that have led to discrimination against healthy members of high-risk groups, to parental abandonment of young AIDS victims, and to consideration of quarantine laws in municipalities throughout the country. These fears and their effects on the population are similar in many respects to those generated by past epidemics. Consider this perceptive description of an outbreak of bubonic plague during the Napoleonic campaigns of 1798 to 1801 in Egypt and Syria:

> To the list of the three contending powers in Egypt, France, Britain and Turkey, must be added a fourth, bubonic plague, perhaps the most masterful belligerent of all. The Pest could cripple an army by reducing manpower but the greatest danger was fear. In the healthy terror could produce symptoms simulating acute illness; in an infected person it might so influence the course of the disease that death was the inevitable outcome; in the mass, even among disciplined troops, it could bring about a general and profound demoralisation.*

The British naval surgeon quoted above did not have the tools to substantiate his belief that fear influenced the course of disease in individual patients. Today's medical scientists are more fortunate. Investigation of the relationship between stress and immune function in patients infected with HTLV-III/LAV is just one of the areas being pursued by AIDS researchers. Scientists are exploring a wide range of psycho-social issues affecting AIDS patients and their families, healthy members of high-risk groups, health care providers, and the general population.

The AIDS crisis also has generated extremely complex policy issues, discussed further in Chapter 8. The tremendous financial burdens imposed by AIDS are appearing at a time when policymakers at every level of government have called for a reduction in health care spending. Who should pay for clinical and supportive services for AIDS patients? How much

---

*Geoffrey Marks and William K. Beatty, *Epidemics* (New York: Charles Scribner's Sons, 1976), p. 253.

money should be devoted to AIDS research? How should funds be divided among competing research needs? The questions are endless. Enormous effort will be required to develop reasonable and equitable answers.

An equally difficult problem is how to balance the health needs of the community against the civil rights of those who may be carriers of the virus. For example, public health experts have very different views about the reporting of test results that indicate exposure to HTLV-III/LAV. Some believe that mandatory reporting and contact tracing are necessary to slow the spread of the virus. Tracing individuals who have been exposed and offering them serologic screening and risk-reduction education would be especially beneficial in populations with a low prevalence of disease, they say. Others express concern, however, that mandatory reporting might discourage some high-risk persons from taking the test. In fact, some spokesmen within the homosexual community have discouraged other homosexuals from taking the test because of the potential loss of confidentiality. Disagreements grow even sharper over the ethical and moral implications of mandatory testing and the possibility of quarantining AIDS victims who continue to engage in high-risk behavior without concern for the health of others.

Other questions arise over who should be responsible for the production and distribution of educational materials about AIDS both for high-risk groups and the general public. Homosexual communities in large urban areas have used a mix of public and private funds to achieve a high level of awareness about AIDS risk factors among their members. Very little information is available, however, for homosexuals from non-English-speaking minorities or for persons at risk because of drug abuse. Should federal, state, or local governments or private-sector organizations meet these needs?

Some people believe that it is inappropriate for government agencies to tell homosexuals how to have "safe sex" or to explain the importance of sterile needles to drug abusers. Others feel that the gravity of the situation warrants such measures. These conflicts must be resolved as rapidly as possible. Ignoring them will only hamper efforts to slow the spread of infection.

The development of risk-reduction information for the general public is on firmer ground. For example, the American Red Cross announced in late 1985 that it was seeking assistance from others in the private sector to establish the Red Cross AIDS Public Education Program. Building on the strength of the Red Cross national network, this program will provide an extensive array of educational activities and information for community organizations, health care professionals, corporate and business leaders, and public officials. These efforts will supplement programs funded through the Public Health Service and by state and local governments.

The importance of widespread public understanding of the AIDS crisis cannot be overemphasized. This book is designed to provide an accessible overview of the scientific facts and social implications of AIDS as they appear in mid-1986. While every effort has been made to keep pace with new scientific advances and with shifting social and political tides, the field is moving very rapidly, and certain details will no doubt change before the printer's ink dries. That should not detract from the book's principal message: at present, control of the AIDS epidemic depends on education and other public health measures to change high-risk sexual behavior and to reduce the spread of infection among intravenous drug abusers. The serious and complex problems created by the AIDS crisis will be solved only through the cooperation of every segment of American society.

2
Tracking the Epidemic

AIDS is still only a moderately common disease in the United States—as indicated earlier, about 19,000 cases have been reported. But scientists believe that 1 million or more persons have been infected with the virus HTLV-III/LAV. This chapter traces the development of the AIDS epidemic and the dimensions of the disease within specific risk groups.

Transmission of the Virus

It must be emphasized at the outset that there is no evidence that AIDS can be transmitted by "casual" contact. HTLV-III/LAV, the virus that causes AIDS, does not penetrate the skin, the epithelial cells lining the respiratory tract, or the mucosa of the digestive tract. Thus, the disease cannot be transmitted by a handshake, by a cough or sneeze, or by the consumption of food prepared by someone with AIDS. Moderate heat (158° F for 10 minutes), standard solutions of almost all common disinfectants, and an ordinary dilution of household bleach (one part bleach to ten parts water) inactivate HTLV-III/LAV.

Long-term studies of the families of adult and pediatric AIDS patients and of thousands of health care personnel demonstrate that the virus is not transmitted by any daily activity related to living with or caring for an AIDS patient. Siblings of children with AIDS have remained free of infection even after sharing beds and toothbrushes with a sick child.

Fears about the possibility of catching AIDS through casual contact were most intense among the general public shortly after researchers announced that they could isolate the virus from body fluids other than blood and semen. Subsequent studies have shown, however, that the virus is very rare in secretions such as tears and saliva, and even when it is present the levels are probably too low to play a role in infection.

The virus is transmitted when virus particles or infected cells gain direct access to the bloodstream. This can occur during anal intercourse (the receiving partner is at greatest risk), vaginal intercourse (male-to-female transmission has been well documented; some scientists still question the potential for female-to-male transmission*), and probably oral/genital intercourse with an infected partner. The other major routes of transmission involve sharing of needles among intravenous (IV) drug abusers and infected mothers' passing the virus to their unborn or newborn children.

The likelihood of infection appears to depend in part on the quantity of virus transmitted; a small dose probably cannot withstand normal body defense mechanisms. This would explain the rarity of infection among health care workers who accidentally stick themselves with infected needles.

Finally, studies of women whose husbands or sexual partners are infected with HTLV-III/LAV indicate that some individuals may be more resistant to the virus than others. The reasons for this apparent difference are not yet clear. Genetic factors may play a role, and recent laboratory studies suggest that health status also may be important. These studies show that certain components of the immune system are most susceptible to infection with HTLV-III/LAV when they are actively engaged in fighting other kinds of infections.

---

*In March 1986, researchers in both Boston and San Francisco reported that they had isolated HTLV-III/LAV from cervical secretions of women who had HTLV-III/LAV antibodies in their blood. These findings suggest that female genital secretions may be a source for sexual transmission of the virus to men. Support for female-to-male transmission appeared in a letter, "Transmission of HTLV-III Infection from Man to Woman to Man," in the *New England Journal of Medicine*, April 10, 1986, p. 987.

These facts convey several important messages:

1. Indiscriminate sex with multiple partners may increase the risk of contracting AIDS for heterosexuals as well as homosexuals, because it increases the likelihood of engaging in sexual activity with someone carrying the virus.

2. Everyone should know the infection status of his or her sexual partners; those who are not infected should avoid intercourse with those who are infected.

3. Condoms should be used in any sexual encounter not part of a long-term stable relationship. Although condoms have not been proved effective in limiting the transmission of AIDS, they have been shown to prevent passage of HTLV-III/LAV in the laboratory, and they reduce the spread of other sexually transmitted diseases.

4. Women who are members of high-risk groups or whose partners may be infected should postpone pregnancy until more is known about the disease. Women who appear healthy can transmit the virus to their babies before birth and immediately after birth, perhaps through breast feeding.

5. Members of known high-risk groups should not donate blood, blood products, organs, tissues, or semen.

Development of the Epidemic

When the first cases of AIDS were reported in 1981, epidemiologists at the Centers for Disease Control in Atlanta immediately began tracking the disease, backward in time as well as forward. They determined that the first cases of AIDS in the United States probably occurred in 1977.

By early 1982 AIDS had appeared in 15 states, the District of Columbia, and 2 foreign countries, but the total number of cases remained low: 158 men and 1 woman. More than 90 percent of the men were homosexual or bisexual. Interviews with patients did not provide any definite clues about the origin of the disease.

Then in July 1982 the CDC published a report from the University of Miami describing unusual infections and Kaposi's sarcoma in 34 recent Haitian immigrants (including four women) in five states. The authors of the report noted the similarities between this new phenomenon and the pattern of disease previously described in homosexual men and intravenous drug abusers. None of the Haitian men reported homosexual activity, however, and only one had a history of intravenous drug abuse. (The difficulties associated with cross-cultural studies of disease transmission are described later in this section.) These findings led to speculation that AIDS might have been introduced into the U.S. homosexual community by men who had contracted the disease while vacationing in Haiti. It soon became clear, however, that the syndrome also was new in that country.

The puzzling report about the Haitian patients was followed immediately by news that AIDS had appeared in three heterosexual men with hemophilia. Together, these reports provided strong support for the theory that the syndrome was caused by an infectious agent. They also weakened the conviction that AIDS was overwhelmingly a disease of homosexuals.

The potential magnitude of the AIDS problem became clear in 1983. By December of that year, 3,000 cases of AIDS had been reported in adults from 42 states, the District of Columbia, and Puerto Rico, and the disease had been recognized in 20 other countries. Researchers had identified cases suggesting transmission from mother to unborn baby and through blood transfusions. The risk group pattern began to take on many of the characteristics still observed today: 71 percent of cases involved homosexual or bisexual men and 17 percent involved men and women who abused intravenous drugs. Of the remaining patients, 5 percent were Haitian immigrants, 1 percent were hemophiliacs, 1 percent were heterosexual partners of men or women in high-risk groups, and 1 percent were transfusion recipients. About 4 percent did not fit into any known risk category.

The relentless increase in total cases continued through 1984 and 1985 (see Figure 3). By the end of December 1985, the number of reported cases had risen to almost 16,000.

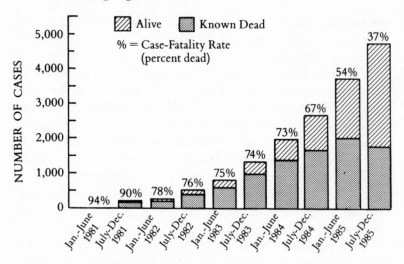

FIGURE 3.   Reported cases of AIDS and case-fatality rates in the United States, by date of first report to the Centers for Disease Control, 1981 through 1985. Bottom (dotted) portion of bar indicates number of cases in each half-year group known dead as of April 4, 1986. Source: U.S. Department of Health and Human Services, Public Health Service, Centers for Disease Control.

The Incidence of AIDS in the United States

As of April 4, 1986, physicians and health departments in the United States had notified the CDC of 19,181 AIDS patients (18,907 adults and 274 children), of whom 10,152 had died. Among the adult AIDS patients, 60 percent were white, 25 percent were black, and 14 percent were Hispanic. Ninety-four percent were men.

The distribution of cases classified by recognized risk factors for AIDS has remained relatively constant:

- 73 percent in homosexual or bisexual men
- 17 percent in intravenous drug abusers
- 1 percent in persons with hemophilia
- 1 percent in heterosexual sex partners of high-risk persons
- 2 percent in blood transfusion recipients

The proportion of AIDS patients classified as not belonging to a recognized risk group also has remained constant, at about 6 percent. This category includes recent Haitian immigrants and others born in countries in which most AIDS cases have not been associated with known risk factors.

The chances of contracting AIDS for those who are not members of a recognized risk group remain extremely low: less than one in a million. But some groups have been hit very hard. The population-specific annual incidence rates of AIDS among single men in Manhattan and San Francisco, intravenous drug abusers in New York City and New Jersey, and persons with hemophilia A are between 260 and 350 per 100,000—close to the incidence of cancer among the general population in the United States.

Another way to view this risk is to consider the effect of AIDS on the life expectancies of members of high-risk groups. One standard measure of premature mortality is "years of potential life lost" (YPLL) before age 65. In 1980 the most common causes of YPLL for single (never married) men between 25 and 44 years of age were automobile and other accidents, murder and suicide, and cancer. Only four years later, AIDS was responsible for more YPLL in young single men in Manhattan than any other factor; in San Francisco it had surpassed all other causes of YPLL combined.

AIDS also has caused a dramatic increase in the total YPLL in this high-risk population. In 1984 the YPLL among single men aged 25 to 44 increased by 5 percent nationwide, by 43 percent in Manhattan, and by almost 75 percent in San Francisco.

The International Incidence of AIDS

The proportion of AIDS cases attributed to heterosexual contact, homosexual contact, intravenous drug abuse, and other modes of transmission varies considerably among countries, for reasons that are not completely understood. Further study of these differences may provide important clues about factors that increase or decrease susceptibility to infection with HTLV-III/LAV.

Europe   The incidence of AIDS in most European countries is considerably lower than that in the United States, but transmission appears to be accelerating. During 1984 an average of 10 new cases was diagnosed each week in Europe; in contrast, the average number of new cases per week by September 1985 was 27. (At that time, about 125 new cases were reported each week in the United States.) The highest rates were reported in Switzerland and Denmark, each with slightly more than 1 case per 100,000 population. Belgium had a similar rate, but 72 percent of its cases originated in equatorial Africa.

As in the United States, male homosexuals account for the highest percentage of European AIDS cases (69 percent). Several 1985 studies indicate that HTLV-III/LAV infection has begun to spread rapidly among intravenous drug users in Europe. Of the 1,573 European AIDS cases reported by September 1985, 8 percent were among drug abusers, compared with 2 percent of 421 cases reported by July 1984. More than 40 percent of the cases in Italy and Spain have occurred in this group.

Africa   In central Africa, the AIDS problem has become extremely serious. In Zaire, for example, the minimum incidence of the syndrome has been calculated at 17 cases per 100,000 population (contrasted with about 6 cases per 100,000 in the United States). Preliminary studies indicate that between 5 and 10 percent of the population of central Africa may be infected with HTLV-III/LAV.

One of the first warning signs of this crisis was the appearance of an unusually virulent form of Kaposi's sarcoma, similar to that seen in AIDS patients in the United States. Unlike the classic form of this cancer (which is widespread in Africa), atypical Kaposi's sarcoma invades the digestive tract and the lungs and is very difficult to treat. Studies in Uganda and Zambia have shown that this aggressive disease is strongly associated with HTLV-III/LAV infection.

A new wasting syndrome called slim disease, first described in Uganda, also has been linked to HTLV-III/LAV and is now believed to be another form of AIDS. Victims of this syndrome have severe diarrhea and extreme weight loss (usually more than 20 pounds). They also may exhibit some of the opportunistic infections characteristic of AIDS. There is no treatment for this disease, and most of the men, women, and children affected die within a year.

The pattern of AIDS in central Africa is different in many respects from that in the United States. Almost half of African AIDS patients are women. Also, several studies have found an association between infection with HTLV-III/LAV in central Africa and heterosexual promiscuity, especially involving female prostitution. For example, a 1984 study of blood samples from a small group of prostitutes in Butare, Rwanda, showed a very high level of exposure to the virus (antibodies to HTLV-III/LAV were found in 29 of 33 prostitutes tested). In the same study, 7 of 25 men treated for sexually transmitted diseases who admitted having contact with prostitutes also tested positive. In contrast, exposure to the virus among a control group was 12 percent for women and 7 percent for men.

These and other facts have led some researchers to conclude that heterosexual contact is the dominant mode of transmission of HTLV-III/LAV in central Africa. Other scientists are less certain, pointing out the extreme difficulty of conducting cross-cultural studies of disease transmission. Unsanitary health practices, such as reuse of hypodermic needles, and ritual practices that involve cutting and scarring with unsterile instruments also could contribute to the high incidence of AIDS among men, women, and children. In addition, social mores and distrust of foreign interviewers may interfere with efforts to assess the likelihood of known high-risk sexual behaviors. For example, in cultures that have very strong prohibitions against homosexuality, men may be unwilling to report sexual contacts with other men.

An alternative explanation for the high incidence of infection among promiscuous heterosexual men in these countries is that they are more likely than other men to develop a whole range of sexually transmitted diseases, and therefore are more likely to seek treatment from folk-medicine practitioners using contaminated needles. The same is true of prostitutes, who also are at increased risk of infection because of contacts with bisexual men.

There is an urgent need for more information about the modes of transmission of HTLV-III/LAV in Africa, and about possible cofactors that increase the risk of disease among those infected with the virus.

Haiti   The distribution of AIDS cases in Haiti has many features in common with that in central Africa, although the overall incidence of disease is much lower (the total number of cases in Haiti was 363 in January 1986). Few of the cases have been traced to homosexuality or drug abuse, and 30 percent of AIDS victims are women. Haiti became a focal point of AIDS research because of the high incidence of disease among recent Haitian immigrants to the United States. Haitian immigrants were classified by the CDC as a separate risk group for AIDS until July 1985, when epidemiologists concluded that unique risk factors could not be identified among Haitians.

Medical records in Haiti indicate that AIDS appeared in that country at about the same time it appeared in the United States, in early 1978. Jean Pape of the Haitian Study Group on Kaposi's Sarcoma and Opportunistic Infections and his colleagues reported in an early paper on AIDS that a large proportion of Haitian cases originated in Carrefour, known as a center of male and female prostitution. Patients also had a high incidence of other venereal infections, again suggesting a correlation between the disease and indiscriminate sexual activity.

The differences between AIDS risk factors in developing countries and in industrialized nations present an important area for further study. Researchers are particularly interested in the impact of environmental factors and other diseases, such as tuberculosis and malaria, on the natural history of HTLV-III/LAV infection. Understanding why the syndrome spreads faster or slower and by different routes in various populations will be crucial for worldwide control of AIDS.

(International travelers should use caution when seeking medical care in foreign countries. While prevention of AIDS transmission through blood transfusion is now effective in most European countries, this is not the case in many other parts of the world. Also, in many developing countries medications are given primarily by injection, often in local pharmacies or clinics—travelers should be wary of unsterile syringes and other contaminated equipment in such settings.)

Recognizing the Extent of Infection

The first cases of AIDS in the United States led medical scientists to take a closer look at the health of the rest of the homosexual community. Physicians had known for many years that homosexual men who reported large numbers of sexual partners had more episodes of venereal disease and were at higher risk of hepatitis B infection than the rest of the population, but coincidentally with the appearance of AIDS, other debilitating problems began to appear more frequently.

The most common was chronic generalized lymphade-nopathy (swollen glands), often accompanied by extreme fatigue, weight loss, fever, chronic diarrhea, mild immune-system abnormalities, decreased levels of blood platelets (cells that prevent excessive bleeding), and fungal infections in the mouth. This condition was labeled AIDS-related complex, or ARC. Some ARC patients remained stable indefinitely. Others developed AIDS.

Researchers suspected that AIDS, ARC, and a range of milder aberrations of the immune system probably represented different responses to the same infectious agent. The possibility that some persons without symptoms might be capable of transmitting the infection was suggested by several cases of transfusion-associated AIDS, in which the donors had appeared healthy at the time of blood donation but later developed signs of ARC or AIDS.

The isolation of HTLV-III/LAV in 1983 and 1984 and the development of techniques to produce large quantities of the virus paved the way for a battery of tests to determine the relationship between AIDS and ARC and the magnitude of the carrier problem.

Antibody Tests

The first priority after isolation of the virus was to verify its association with the diseases in question. Using several different laboratory tests, scientists looked for antibodies (proteins produced by the immune system in response to infection) against HTLV-III/LAV in the blood of AIDS and ARC patients. They found that almost 100 percent of AIDS patients and more than 90 percent of ARC patients had the antibodies—they were seropositive. In contrast, less than 1 percent of persons with no known risk factors were seropositive.

The next step was to look for antibodies in people from high-risk groups who appeared healthy. Researchers were surprised by the large numbers of risk-group members who tested positive. Studies showed that the rates of seropositivity were between 22 percent and 65 percent for homosexual men (men who had more sexual partners were more likely to be positive); 87 percent for intravenous drug abusers admitted to a detoxification program in New York City; between 56 percent and 72 percent for patients with hemophilia A (patients who required more clotting factor tended to have higher seropositivity rates); and 35 percent for women who were sexual partners of men with AIDS.

What do these high seropositivity rates mean? Scientists know part of the answer, but they will need more time to piece together the full story.

The presence of specific antibodies in the blood against viruses that cause acute diseases such as measles shows that a previous infection registered on the body's immune system or that a vaccine elicited an appropriate antibody response. The antibody molecules that remain in the bloodstream are like scouts: if the virus appears again, the scouts recognize it immediately and prevent it from gaining a foothold. Thus, people rarely develop measles a second time, although they may encounter the measles virus hundreds of times after initial exposure. In many infectious diseases, such as polio, a person can develop protective antibodies against the causative agent without showing any signs of disease.

HTLV-III/LAV produces a chronic viral infection. The antibodies do not seem to correlate with elimination of the virus. Harold Jaffe of the Centers for Disease Control and his colleagues were able to isolate active virus from the blood of 12 out of 20 homosexual men who had antibodies but no symptoms for between two and six years. Robert C. Gallo of the National Cancer Institute and his co-workers report that they can isolate virus from the blood of more than 80 percent of people with detectable antibodies.

These findings mean that most, if not all, people who have antibodies against HTLV-III/LAV carry active virus. Until proved otherwise, these individuals should be considered infectious. However, they are infectious only through sexual practices that involve an exchange of body fluids, through shared intravenous needles, and, for women, through transmission to their unborn or breastfed children.

Individual Risk After Infection

Using data from San Francisco, federal officials estimate that between 5 and 10 percent of those infected with HTLV-III/LAV will develop AIDS within two to five years, but some populations of infected persons seem to have a higher incidence of disease than others. For example, two studies of infected homosexual men in New York City found AIDS rates of 25 percent and 34 percent after less than four years of study. Several factors could explain this wide variation. Participants in the New York studies may have been infected with HTLV-III/LAV longer than those in the San Francisco study.

Another possible explanation is that certain "cofactors" (such as other viral infections or drug use) may increase the risk of developing AIDS. Many researchers believe that identification of potential cofactors could help reduce the incidence of disease.

In addition to those who develop AIDS, another 25 percent of those infected with HTLV-III/LAV may develop ARC within two to five years, according to the CDC study of homosexual men in San Francisco. The outlook for ARC patients remains unclear: early reports indicated that between 6 and 20 percent would develop AIDS (see Chapter 3 for fuller discussion of this issue). ARC patients who are sick enough to require medical care early in the course of their disease appear to be more likely to progress to AIDS.

The critical question in making long-term predictions about AIDS is whether an infected person's risk of getting sick will decrease as the years pass. Scientists hope at some point to be able to tell patients, "If you don't develop AIDS within five years [or six, seven, or eight years, depending on the results of ongoing studies], then you are unlikely to get it at all." So far, there is no evidence of decreasing risk over time, but experience with the disease is very limited. If the risk proves not to drop over time, then the overall incidence of disease among infected persons may be much higher than originally expected.

Recent clinical reports and new evidence of HTLV-III/LAV in the brain indicate that this virus also causes debilitating neurological disease. Chapter 4 explores the relationship between HTLV-III/LAV and viruses that cause slow but progressive brain infections and other symptoms in sheep, goats, horses, and probably monkeys. The similarities between these viruses and the one that causes AIDS suggest an even more disturbing question: How many of those who withstand the assault of HTLV-III/LAV on the immune system will eventually succumb to its effects on the brain?

These issues demonstrate the importance to the individual of avoiding infection with HTLV-III/LAV through sensible health practices, such as those mentioned earlier in this chapter. They also underscore the urgency of developing new methods to help those already infected.

Societal Implications

While CDC epidemiologists estimate that 1 million or more Americans have been infected with HTLV-III/LAV, other researchers believe that the total may be closer to 2 million. This uncertainty reflects the need for more information about the natural history of HTLV-III/LAV infection. The long lag time between infection and the appearance of clinical symptoms hampers efforts to determine the prevalence of infection nationally and also makes it difficult for communities with low levels of AIDS to appreciate the magnitude of the AIDS-related problems they could face in the future. James W. Curran, chief of the AIDS Branch at CDC, says that in many areas the number of persons infected with HTLV-III/LAV is at least 100 times the number with AIDS. Thus, education and planning must begin before the disease is widespread, or preventive efforts will come too late.

If a large proportion of those infected eventually become sick, the disease could exert a major impact on the nation's economy. Researchers estimate that between $42,000 and $147,000 is spent for the hospital care of each AIDS patient. Expenditures could be reduced by increasing the availability of outpatient and community services, but few communities have taken the steps necessary to develop these programs (see Chapter 8).

High-Risk Groups and Unexplained Cases

This section focuses on the incidence and spread of AIDS within specific high-risk groups and then reviews adult AIDS cases that have not been classified by recognized risk factors. Pediatric AIDS is examined separately.

Homosexual Men

According to CDC's Curran, one of the most insidious barriers to the development of a rational approach to AIDS is fatalism among homosexuals and health care providers about its impact—especially the belief that all homosexual men will become infected and that many of them will die.

Curran estimates that the incidence of infection among homosexual men in the United States is still less than 30 percent. The challenge for the individual homosexual man to remain uninfected is difficult but not impossible. Cities throughout the world report a decline in other sexually transmitted infections—particularly gonorrhea—among homosexual men, indicating that many are having fewer sexual encounters. In areas where the prevalence of HTLV-III/LAV infection is still low, this precaution could make a difference.

Unfortunately, in San Francisco and some other U.S. coastal cities, the positive effects of recommended behavior changes have been at least partially counterbalanced by increased numbers of men infected with HTLV-III/LAV. Between 1980 and 1984 the incidence of rectal gonorrhea among men in San Francisco fell from 5,000 cases to about 1,300 cases, a drop of 73 percent. At the same time, however, the prevalence of HTLV-III/LAV antibody in a study group of homosexual men increased from 24 percent to 68 percent. Statistically, if a man had 12 partners from that study group in 1980, on average he would have been exposed to 3 men infected with HTLV-III/LAV. If by 1984 he had only 3 sexual partners (a reduction of 75 percent), 2 of the 3 could have been infected because of the increased prevalence of infection. Thus, a substantial change in behavior did not produce a concomitant reduction in risk.

Reducing the number of sexual partners may have other benefits, however. Researchers at the National Cancer Institute and the New England Deaconess Hospital in Boston found that infected but healthy homosexual men who had more than six sexual partners annually were more likely to have active virus particles in their blood than infected men who had fewer sexual partners. The presence of virus particles might make such men more infectious to others and at greater risk of developing disease themselves. Thus, avoiding indiscriminate sexual encounters may be as important for those with HTLV-III/LAV antibodies as it is for those without antibodies. In any sexual encounters with partners who may be infected, care should be taken to avoid the exchange of blood, semen, and other body fluids.

Many factors probably contributed to the rapid transmission of HTLV-III/LAV once it entered the homosexual population. Among them were the tendency toward large numbers of sexual partners, sexual practices that carried a high risk of abrading delicate tissues (increasing the likelihood of virus entering the bloodstream), and immune systems impaired by numerous previous infections with other viruses, bacteria, and parasites.

Intravenous Drug Abusers

Intravenous drug abusers constitute 65 percent of all heterosexual AIDS patients. Thus, this group is a major factor in the dissemination of HTLV-III/LAV to the heterosexual population.

Nationwide, the population-specific annual incidence rate of AIDS among IV drug abusers is about 168 per 100,000, but the rates in New York City and New Jersey exceed 260 per 100,000 (reported in 1985). These two geographical areas account for almost 70 percent of AIDS cases among drug abusers. The majority of these cases occur in men, in part because men have a higher incidence of drug abuse. When AIDS cases in homosexual or bisexual male IV drug abusers are excluded, the rate in men remains 1.5 to 1.8 times higher than that in women.

Needle sharing and the practice in some "shooting galleries" of drawing blood back into the syringe before injecting a drug are the likely sources of AIDS transmission among IV drug abusers. This is a very difficult group in which to implement behavior changes. One alternative suggested by some public health officials is to provide free or low-cost sterile injection equipment. The controversy surrounding this issue is discussed in Chapter 6.

Some researchers believe that intravenous drug abuse among female prostitutes in the United States may be a major source of transmission of HTLV-III/LAV to the heterosexual population. This assumes that female-to-male transmission is at least moderately efficient.

Hemophiliacs

Almost 1 percent of persons with hemophilia A in the United States have been diagnosed with AIDS (155 cases), and more than 80 percent have antibodies against HTLV-III/LAV. The one bright note is that new procedures for inactivating the virus in the blood products used to treat hemophilia have eliminated this risk factor for hemophiliacs diagnosed in the future.

Hemophiliacs lack one of several blood proteins required for normal clotting. The most common form of the disease is hemophilia A, caused by an inability to manufacture the antihemophilia factor, or factor VIII; patients with hemophilia B lack another clotting factor, called factor IX. Prior to the development of techniques to extract factor VIII and factor IX concentrates from human plasma (plasma is the liquid part of the blood), these patients endured frequent bleeding and some were in danger of fatal bleeding episodes.

Conventional methods of manufacturing these concentrates placed the hemophiliac population at high risk of infection with HTLV-III/LAV. The concentrates are extracted from pooled plasma obtained from thousands of donors. Unlike some other blood products, such as albumin, the concentrates could not be pasteurized, because heat inactivated the clotting factors. Plasma from one infected donor could contaminate the entire pool and thereby transmit the virus to many hemophiliacs.

In the fall of 1984, several laboratories announced new methods of protecting the clotting factors from high temperatures. With these techniques, manufacturers can heat the pooled blood fractions sufficiently to inactivate HTLV-III/LAV and still retain the clotting function. All hemophiliacs in the United States now use the heat-treated products.

The cumulative incidence of AIDS and AIDS-related

conditions among infected recipients of clotting factor—between 2 and 4 percent—is lower than the cumulative incidence among infected homosexuals. The reasons for this difference are not known. Several more years must pass before scientists know how infection will affect those now free of symptoms—whether they will remain healthy or whether the current figures indicate a very long lag time with a bleak outlook.

One study suggests the possibility of progressive disruption of the immune system in these patients. Researchers following hemophiliacs who developed antibodies to HTLV-III/LAV over a five-year span found that 70 percent of those who had been seropositive for more than three years had lymphadenopathy, compared with 10 percent of those who had been seropositive three years or less. The first group also had a higher incidence of other immune-system abnormalities.

Heterosexual Sex Partners of High-Risk Individuals

Almost two-thirds of the 257 cases (April 4, 1986) in this category involve the sexual partners of intravenous drug abusers, but cases also have been reported among the female partners of hemophiliacs and bisexual men. In fact, only 45 of the individuals in this group are men.

One explanation for the small number of men in this category is that AIDS is more readily transmitted by men to their female partners than vice versa. Other possible explanations are that there are still relatively few women with AIDS in the population capable of transmitting the virus, or that the partners of female drug abusers are more likely to be drug abusers themselves and therefore would be counted in that high-risk group.

Unexplained Cases

Unexplained cases of AIDS in adults are those not traced to homosexuality, intravenous drug abuse, receipt of blood or blood products, or sexual intercourse with a member of a recognized high-risk group. CDC researchers reviewed the origins of cases in the "unexplained" category in a report issued on January 17, 1986. Of the 984 cases in the category at that time, 398 involved persons born outside the United States (primarily Haitians). The incidence of AIDS among recent Haitian immigrants has not increased as rapidly as that among the groups at highest risk. While the total number of AIDS cases increased by 89 percent in 1985, the number of cases among Haitian immigrants increased by only 25 percent.

The remaining 586 unexplained cases included 297 that were still under investigation and 178 in which information on patients was incomplete (owing to death, refusal to be interviewed, or loss to follow-up). In interviews with the 111 patients for whom no risk factor could be identified after follow-up, 39 had histories of gonorrhea or syphilis; 15 of the 57 men interviewed reported sexual contact with a female prostitute. These facts suggest a possible association between a small number of AIDS cases and heterosexual promiscuity in this country.

The principal studies on heterosexual transmission of HTLV-III/LAV in the United States were reported by Robert Redfield of the Walter Reed Army Institute of Research in Washington, D.C., and his colleagues. Of 41 sequential cases of AIDS or ARC evaluated at the Walter Reed Army Medical Center by these researchers, 15 (10 men and 5 women) appeared to involve heterosexual transmission. Heterosexual contact with high-risk partners was documented in 6 of the 15 cases. The other 9 patients reported multiple sexual partners (more than 50) or sexual contact with prostitutes. The researchers concluded that their observations provided epidemiologic evidence supporting the occurrence of bidirectional heterosexual transmission (both male to female and female to male) of HTLV-III/LAV infection and disease.

Scientists who disagree with this conclusion (especially as regards female-to-male transmission) say that the military's punitive stance on intravenous drug abuse and homosexual activity might have discouraged the soldiers from admitting that they had been involved in such high-risk activities. They note that even if these cases do represent heterosexual trans-

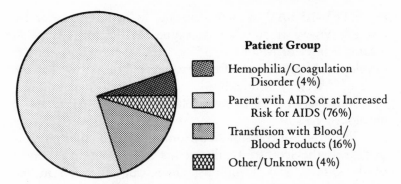

FIGURE 4.   Distribution of pediatric AIDS cases (total = 274) in the United States: percentage by patient group, 1981 through April 4, 1986. Source: U.S. Department of Health and Human Services, Public Health Service, Centers for Disease Control.

mission, Redfield's report should not be taken as an indication of growing heterosexual transmission within the general population, because military personnel tend to have a disproportionate number of all sexually transmitted diseases.

Until more research has been done to determine the true risk of female-to-male transmission, heterosexual men as well as heterosexual women should assume that indiscriminate sexual activity is high-risk behavior, especially in areas where the incidence of HTLV-III/LAV infection is highest.

Children at Risk

In the United States more than 270 children under 13 years of age have been diagnosed with AIDS, and more than half of them have died. As shown in Figure 4, three-quarters of these children come from families in which one or both parents have AIDS or are at increased risk of developing AIDS. Most of the remaining pediatric patients are hemophiliacs or recipients of multiple transfusions. About 4 percent of AIDS cases in children have been unexplained, and most are awaiting further epidemiologic information about the parents. Even women who appear completely healthy can transmit HTLV-III/LAV to their offspring. In a study reported by Gwendolyn Scott and her colleagues at the University of Miami School of Medicine, 15 of 16 mothers whose infants developed AIDS shortly after birth were clinically well at the time of delivery, although all had some abnormal immune functions. Five of these women later developed AIDS and 7 developed ARC.

The mode of transmission from mother to child remains unclear. In the Scott study, the infants' average age at the onset of the disease was 4 months, suggesting infection in the womb, during delivery, or shortly after birth. Support for transmission in the womb (as opposed to transmission involving passage through the vagina at birth) comes from a case described by Canadian physicians, who found evidence of HTLV-III/LAV infection in an infant delivered by caesarean section from a mother who died with AIDS two hours later. A report by Australian scientists indicates that infants also can be infected after birth, probably through breast milk; they describe AIDS in an infant whose mother developed antibodies to HTLV-III/LAV following a postpartum transfusion.

The U.S. Public Health Service recommends that women who believe they might have been exposed to HTLV-III/LAV postpone pregnancy until more is known about the syndrome. In high-risk communities, physicians should consider making the antibody test for HTLV-III/LAV part of a complete prepregnancy or prenatal screening program.

Groups Not at High Risk

Questions arise frequently about two other population groups that might appear to be at high risk of AIDS: homosexual women and health care providers.

Homosexual Women

Homosexual women tend to have a very low incidence of venereal disease in general, and AIDS is no exception. There are no reported cases of transmission of HTLV-III/LAV through female homosexual contact.

Health Care Workers

The few apparent work-related infections with HTLV-III/LAV among health care personnel have involved needle sticks or other puncture wounds with equipment previously used on AIDS patients. There is no evidence of airborne spread of the virus or of interpersonal spread through casual contact. Thus, health care workers who avoid accidents such as those mentioned appear to be at no greater risk of infection than the general population.

In some hospitals the incidence of accidental injuries with potentially contaminated instruments is surprisingly high. In a study of such accidents among health care workers, Stanley Weiss of the National Cancer Institute and his colleagues found that 35 of 239 house staff officers (physicians in training) and 4 of 39 laboratory workers in a major metropolitan hospital reported at least one possible percutaneous exposure to HTLV-III/LAV, usually injuries with needles that had been used on AIDS patients. Fortunately, a single incident of this type appears to carry a very low risk of infection. Studies of almost 1,000 health care workers followed after a needle stick or similar injury have identified only 2 cases in which workers not belonging to a known high-risk group had antibodies against HTLV-III/LAV.

Despite this low incidence of infection from a single puncture wound, the serious consequences of becoming infected with this virus make it essential for all medical personnel to understand and practice proper techniques of drawing blood and handling other body fluids. (See Appendix B for Public Health Service guidelines for health care workers.)

Dental care personnel also should follow precautions to avoid accidental exposure to potentially infective materials. These precautions include the use of gloves, masks, and protective eyewear when performing dental or oral surgical procedures on (1) AIDS patients; (2) members of high-risk groups who have a history of chronic swollen glands, unexplained weight loss, or prolonged fever; (3) hospital patients suspected of having AIDS; and (4) persons known to be infected with HTLV-III/LAV. Instruments used in the mouths of these patients should be sterilized after use. Routine sterilization procedures destroy the HTLV-III/LAV virus, and thus subsequent patients are not at risk of infection.

Reducing the Risk of Transfusion-Associated AIDS

The 299 cases of transfusion-associated AIDS represent about 2 percent of all reported adult cases. The risk of acquiring AIDS from a blood transfusion has never been high. In January 1985, CDC researchers estimated that the incidence of AIDS among adult transfusion recipients during the previous year was about 1 in 250,000 recipients. Recent efforts to increase the safety of the blood supply have reduced this risk considerably.

The possibility that AIDS could be transmitted by blood and blood products was recognized just 18 months after the first reports of the syndrome in the medical literature. The first victims of transfusion-associated AIDS were infants and elderly surgery patients.

In January 1983 the American Red Cross, the American Association of Blood Banks, and the Council of Community Blood Centers issued a joint statement advising their members against accepting donors from known high-risk groups. Intravenous drug abusers and recent Haitian immigrants already were proscribed from blood donation (the latter because they recently had been in a country with endemic malaria), and thus the effect of this statement was to discourage donation by homosexual and bisexual men. Blood service organizations also were urged to screen donors for signs and symptoms of AIDS and to recommend increased reliance on autologous transfusion (by which patients receive their own blood, donated several weeks before an elective surgical procedure). In September 1985 the donor-exclusion criteria were revised to include all men who reported any homosexual encounter after 1977.

Exclusion of high-risk donors was the first phase of a triple attack on the AIDS problem. The second phase involved the implementation of tests to screen blood for laboratory evidence of infection with HTLV-III/LAV, and the third phase was the development of new techniques to inactivate the virus in some blood products. Neither of the last two tasks could have been accomplished, however, if researchers had not worked so quickly to isolate the virus and confirm its association with AIDS and related conditions (see Chapter 4).

The licensing and systemwide adoption of commercial screening tests for HTLV-III/LAV antibodies less than a year after confirmation of the cause of AIDS was a monumental achievement by scientists inside and outside the government and by industry, regulatory agencies, and the blood services complex.

The screening tests use a process called enzyme-linked immunosorbent assay (ELISA). Laboratory technicians begin the ELISA test with a plastic sheet or plastic beads covered with an extremely thin layer of viral proteins (see Figure 5). These proteins are produced by purifying inactivated virus grown in tissue culture. When serum from a prospective blood donor is added to this system, any antibodies made against HTLV-III/LAV stick to the proteins on the sheet. Several steps later, a color reaction indicates whether or not antibodies are present. Reactions are read with a spectrophotometer and graded to indicate the strength of any positive results.

The ELISA tests are not perfect: in populations with a low incidence of infection, the proportion of false positives (positive results in people who do not have antibodies against HTLV-III/LAV) is relatively high. Between March and September of 1985, 2,583,805 units of donated blood were tested by the American Red Cross Blood Services. Of the units tested, 1 percent (25,553 donors) were initially positive. One-quarter of 1 percent (6,345) were positive on a second ELISA test; however, less than 20 percent (985) of those were positive on a more specific test called Western blot analysis.

Community and regional blood centers and hospital blood banks may differ somewhat on the protocols used for AIDS tests, but all have two features in common: (1) blood products that are repeatably reactive on the ELISA are removed from the blood pool, and (2) donors are not notified

TESTING FOR ANTIBODIES TO HTLV-III/LAV

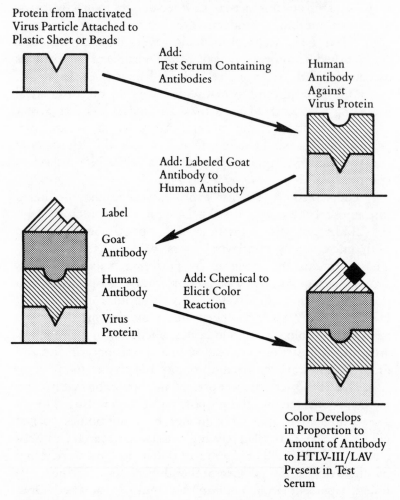

Protein from Inactivated
Virus Particle Attached to
Plastic Sheet or Beads

Add:
Test Serum Containing
Antibodies

Human
Antibody
Against
Virus Protein

Add: Labeled Goat
Antibody to
Human Antibody

Label

Goat
Antibody

Human
Antibody

Add: Chemical to
Elicit Color
Reaction

Virus
Protein

Color Develops
in Proportion to
Amount of Antibody
to HTLV-III/LAV
Present in Test
Serum

FIGURE 5.   Schematic diagram of enzyme-linked immunosorbent assay
(ELISA), process used in commercial screening tests for HTLV-III/LAV
antibodies. Source: Adapted, with permission, from "Sharper Tests for
AIDS," *New Scientist*, Vol. 106, No. 1454 (May 2, 1985), p. 23.

unless subsequent confirmatory tests are also positive. These practices ensure the maximum possible safety of the blood supply and also avoid unnecessary anguish for those who may test positive initially but later are found not to have AIDS antibodies. Most centers also follow Public Health Service guidelines for notifying donors about confirmed positive results (see Figure 6).

The reasons for the false positive tests are not known, but a joint study by the CDC and the Atlanta Red Cross indicates that the majority of those who have a false positive result are women who are slightly older than the average blood donor. Scientists believe that these women may have antibodies against contaminants in the test materials. These contaminants probably are fragments of white blood cells from the cell cultures used to propagate the virus.

In contrast, 93 percent of those with true positive results in the Atlanta study were men, and many had recognized risk factors for AIDS. Also, almost all of the samples that were graded strongly reactive on repeat ELISA tests were Western blot positive, and a majority of these antibody-positive samples contained detectable virus.

One reason for the relatively high number of false positive ELISA tests is that scientists have designed the tests to minimize the number of false negatives (samples that react negatively on the test but actually contain HTLV-III/LAV antibodies and/or virus). This goal is reasonable given the potentially serious consequences of infection.

CDC tests of the sensitivity of ELISA have been encouraging. (Tests that are highly sensitive have a very low probability of producing false negatives.) One test involved 142 blood samples from apparently healthy homosexual men in San Francisco: 70 were ELISA-negative and 72 were ELISA-positive. All of those who were ELISA-negative tested negative on the Western blot analysis, and no blood samples from these patients contained detectable virus. In contrast, the 72 men who were ELISA-positive all had positive Western blot results, and virus was found in 61 percent of blood samples from this group.

Excerpted from:

Provisional Public Health Service Inter-Agency Recommendations for Screening Donated Blood and Plasma for Antibody to the Virus Causing Acquired Immunodeficiency Syndrome

Notification of Donors

If the repeat ELISA test is positive or if other tests are positive, it is the responsibility of the collection facility to ensure that the donor is notified. The information should be given to the donor by an individual especially aware of the sensitivities involved. At present, the proportion of these seropositive donors who have been infected with HTLV-III is not known. It is, therefore, important to emphasize to the donor that the positive result is a preliminary finding that may not represent true infection. To determine the significance of a positive test, the donor should be referred to a physician for evaluation. The information should be given to the donor in a manner to ensure confidentiality of the results and of the donor's identity.

Maintaining Confidentiality

Physicians, laboratory and nursing personnel, and others should recognize the importance of maintaining confidentiality of positive test results. Disclosure of this information for purposes other than medical or public health could lead to serious consequences for the individual. Screening procedures should be designed with safeguards to protect against unauthorized disclosure. Donors should be given a clear explanation of how information about them will be handled. Facilities should consider developing contingency plans in the event that disclosure is sought through legal process. If donor deferral lists are kept, it is necessary to maintain confidentiality of such lists. Whenever appropriate, as an additional safeguard, donor deferral lists should be general, without indication of the reason for inclusion.

Medical Evaluation

The evaluation might include ELISA testing of a follow-up serum specimen and Western blot testing, if the specimen is positive. Persons who continue to show serologic evidence of HTLV-III infection should be questioned about possible exposure to the virus or possible risk factors for AIDS in the individual or his/her sexual contacts and examined for signs of AIDS or related conditions, such as lymphadenopathy, oral candidiasis, Kaposi's sarcoma, and unexplained weight loss. Additional laboratory studies might include tests for other sexually transmitted diseases, tests of immune function, and where available, tests for the presence of the virus, such as viral culture. Testing for antibodies to HTLV-III in the individual's sexual contacts may also be useful in establishing whether the test results truly represent infection. *(Continued)*

36

RECOMMENDATIONS FOR THE INDIVIDUAL

An individual judged most likely to have an HTLV-III infection should be provided the following information and advice:

1. The prognosis for an individual infected with HTLV-III over the long term is not known. However, data available from studies conducted among homosexual men indicate that most persons will remain infected.
2. Although asymptomatic, these individuals may transmit HTLV-III to others. Regular medical evaluation and follow-up is advised, especially for individuals who develop signs or symptoms suggestive of AIDS.
3. Refrain from donating blood, plasma, body organs, other tissue, or sperm.
4. There is a risk of infecting others by sexual intercourse, sharing of needles, and possibly, exposure of others to saliva through oral-genital contact or intimate kissing. The efficacy of condoms in preventing infection with HTLV-III is unproven, but the consistent use of them may reduce transmission.
5. Toothbrushes, razors, or other implements that could become contaminated with blood should not be shared.
6. Women with a seropositive test, or women whose sexual partner is seropositive, are themselves at increased risk of acquiring AIDS. If they become pregnant, their offspring are also at increased risk of acquiring AIDS.
7. After accidents resulting in bleeding, contaminated surfaces should be cleaned with household bleach freshly diluted 1:10 in water.
8. Devices that have punctured the skin, such as hypodermic and acupuncture needles, should be steam sterilized by autoclave before reuse or safely discarded. Whenever possible, disposable needles and equipment should be used.
9. When seeking medical or dental care for intercurrent illness, these persons should inform those responsible for their care of their positive antibody status so that appropriate evaluation can be undertaken and precautions taken to prevent transmission to others.
10. Testing for HTLV-III antibody should be offered to persons who may have been infected as a result of their contact with seropositive individuals (e.g., sexual partners, persons with whom needles have been shared, infants born to seropositive mothers).

Revised recommendations will be published as additional information becomes available and additional experience is gained with this test.

Reported by Centers for Disease Control; Food and Drug Administration; Alcohol, Drug Abuse, and Mental Health Administration; National Institutes of Health; Health Resources and Services Administration.

FIGURE 6.   Public Health Service guidelines for notifying blood donors of confirmed positive results from antibody testing. Source: U.S. Department of Health and Human Services, Public Health Service, Centers for Disease Control. *Morbidity and Mortality Weekly Report*, No. 34 (Jan. 11, 1985), pp. 1–5.

This does not mean that a false negative result with ELISA is impossible. Several researchers have reported that a small number of infected persons do not make antibodies. Others appear to make antibodies against only one major viral protein; unfortunately, this protein is the one most likely to be inactivated or lost during the purification process used to manufacture the ELISA test kits.

These factors, combined with the discovery that some members of high-risk groups continue to attempt to donate blood, make it essential to maintain careful screening of prospective blood donors and to continue efforts to improve blood tests. Future generations of tests might measure viral proteins in the blood rather than antibodies against the virus.

The third phase in increasing the safety of the blood supply, inactivation of infectious agents, is described in the previous section on hemophiliacs. This approach is not feasible for whole blood or for blood components that are destroyed by heat, but it will make a tremendous difference for future patients dependent on clotting-factor concentrates.

Recent advances in reducing HTLV-III/LAV transmission through the blood supply will not begin to affect the incidence of transfusion-associated AIDS for several years because of the three-to-five-year (or longer) lag time between infection and the appearance of clinical symptoms of AIDS.

The risk of transfusion-associated AIDS has been highest for those who received large numbers of units of blood. An analysis by CDC researchers in early 1985 found that recipients of 10 or more units of blood had an incidence of AIDS about 30 times higher than that of recipients of fewer than 10 units. In addition, infants had a higher incidence of disease than adults. Overall, children under one year old make up only 2 percent of blood transfusion recipients, but in the CDC study they accounted for 20 percent of transfusion-associated AIDS cases. This finding leads to two possible conclusions: either the immature immune system is more susceptible to infection with HTLV-III/LAV or infants develop clinical disease more rapidly than older children and adults, and thus those infected are identified sooner.

Conclusion

AIDS and other disease processes associated with HTLV-III/LAV infection will continue to be a serious problem in the United States for the foreseeable future. Homosexual men, intravenous drug abusers, the sexual partners of those in currently identified risk groups, and infants born to infected mothers will continue to be at greatest risk. Transfusion-associated AIDS and AIDS in hemophiliacs also will continue to occur, although the incidence of these cases eventually will decline as a result of donor–exclusion procedures, the implementation of systemwide testing for HTLV-III/LAV antibodies, and new procedures to inactivate the virus in clotting concentrates.

Researchers disagree about the extent to which the virus will spread in the heterosexual population in the United States. Numerous studies indicate that men can transmit the virus to women, although vaginal intercourse may be a less efficient mode of transmission than anal intercourse. The focus of the disagreement is the likelihood of female–to–male transmission. Scientists who think that the risk of female–to–male transmission is extremely small (primarily because the male genital tract is not an efficient portal of entry for the virus) believe that AIDS will not spread much beyond the current risk groups. Others believe that data from Africa and Haiti indicate a higher probability of female–to–male transmission; they expect a gradual increase in the heterosexual spread of the virus in this country.

Communities with only a few cases of AIDS concentrated in high-risk groups cannot afford to ignore the problem until it becomes worse. In both low- and high-risk areas, 100 people may be infected for every person who shows clinical symptoms of the disease because of the three-to-five-year (or longer) lag time between infection and illness. Education programs and other preventive measures must be imple-

These patients both had AIDS. Their conditions, although more complex than those of most AIDS patients, illustrate the potential effects of HTLV-III/LAV, which overwhelms the body's principal defense mechanisms and also infects brain cells. Other than the brain disease—AIDS encephalopathy—caused directly by HTLV-III/LAV infection, the illnesses that devastate patients with AIDS are not new or unique to the syndrome. Many are found in children with congenital defects of the immune system; others are common in cancer or organ transplant patients whose immune systems have been altered by therapeutic drugs. These infections are "opportunistic" (see Table 1); without the opportunity afforded by a weakened immune system they could not establish themselves in the body.

The unique aspects of AIDS are the frequency with which opportunistic infections occur, the tendency for there to be multiple problems in the same patient, and the consistently poor response of patients to treatment. Therapies that work in other populations often fail in AIDS patients because the body simply cannot help itself. Often, illnesses return as soon as treatment ends. Coping with such treatment failures is very difficult in a society accustomed to the reassuring instruction, "Take this antibiotic until the bottle is empty and you'll be fine."

In AIDS patients as in other sick people, the likelihood of defeating an infection or limiting the spread of cancer increases if treatment is begun early; but in AIDS patients it is very easy to let one problem get out of control while focusing on another. Autopsies show that two-thirds of AIDS patients have two or more complications when they die. (Together, the two patients described above had a total of nine infections and two types of cancer.)

Statistics show that so far the cumulative death rate from AIDS is about 50 percent, but more than 70 percent of those diagnosed before July 1984 have died. No one diagnosed with AIDS has ever recovered, although a few have survived for up to five years.

TABLE 1   Microorganisms Causing Opportunistic Infections in Patients with the Acquired Immune Deficiency Syndrome

	Syndromes
Viruses	
Cytomegalovirus	Encephalitis, chorioretinitis, pneumonia, hepatitis, colitis, adrenalitis, disseminated infection
Herpes simplex virus	Persistent, recurrent, or disseminated skin ulcers
Varicella-zoster	Local, severe, or disseminated infection
Epstein-Barr virus	Lymphoma
Papovavirus-JC	Central nervous system infection
Adenoviruses	Colonization, disseminated infection
Bacteria	
Mycobacterium avium-intracellulare[a]	Disseminated infection, severe gastrointestinal disease, massive intraabdominal lymphadenopathy
Mycobacterium tuberculosis[a]	Adenitis, pulmonary infection, meningitis
Mycobacterium species[a]	Disseminated infection
Nocardia asteroides[a]	Pulmonary-pericardial infection, brain abscess
Salmonella species[a]	Typhoidal syndrome, severe gastroenteritis with bacteremia
Listeria monocytogenes[a]	Bacteremia
Legionella species[a]	Pneumonias, cellulitis
Streptococcus pneumoniae[b]	Pneumonia, bacteremia
Haemophilus influenzae[b]	Pneumonia, bacteremia
Staphylococcus aureus[c]	Bacteremia, skin infections, pneumonia
Clostridium perfringens[c]	Bacteremia
Shigella species[c]	Diarrhea, bacteremia
Parasites	
Pneumocystis carinii	Pneumonia
Toxoplasma gondii	Encephalitis, brain abscess
Cryptosporidium species	Gastroenteritis
Fungi	
Candida species	Oropharyngitis, esophagitis, vaginitis
Cryptococcus neoformans	Meningitis, disseminated infection, pneumonia
Histoplasma capsulatum	Disseminated infection
Aspergillus species	Pneumonia

[a]Commonly take advantage of T-cell defects. (See Chapter 5 for discussion of specific cell defects.)
[b]Commonly take advantage of B-cell defects. (See Chapter 5.)
[c]Not associated with identified cell defect.
SOURCE: Adapted, with permission, from D. Armstrong et al., "Treatment of Infections in Patients with the Acquired Immunodeficiency Syndrome," *Annals of Internal Medicine*, Vol. 103, No. 5 (November 1985), Table 1.

Defining the Syndrome

Discussion of the clinical findings associated with AIDS must begin with the understanding that AIDS is only one outcome of infection with HTLV-III/LAV. When epidemiologists at the Centers for Disease Control in Atlanta defined the syndrome in 1982, they placed clear constraints on the types of cases that would be included:

> CDC defines a case of AIDS as a disease, at least moderately predictive of a defect in cell-mediated immunity, occurring in a person with no known cause for diminished resistance to that disease. Such diseases include KS [Kaposi's sarcoma], PCP [*Pneumocystis carinii* pneumonia], and serious OOI [other opportunistic infections]. Diagnoses are considered to fit the case definition only if based on sufficiently reliable methods (generally histology or culture).*

The OOI category included pneumonia, meningitis, and encephalitis caused by nine different viruses, bacteria, fungi, and protozoa; esophagitis (inflammation of the esophagus) caused by candidiasis, cytomegalovirus, or herpes simplex; progressive brain disease with multiple lesions; chronic inflammation of the intestine caused by protozoan parasites of the genus *Cryptosporidium* (lasting more than four weeks); and unusually persistent herpes simplex infections of the mouth or rectum (lasting more than five weeks).

The purpose of these constraints in defining AIDS was to ensure accurate tracking of the syndrome over time. The CDC scientists acknowledged that this case definition would not include the full spectrum of AIDS manifestations, but they emphasized that a less stringent definition might increase the likelihood that non-AIDS diseases would be included in the count and would be more susceptible to reporting inaccuracies. The CDC case definition of AIDS was updated in August 1985 (see Appendix A) to reflect the role of HTLV-III/LAV in the development of the syndrome, but the new definition also

---

*Morbidity and Mortality Weekly Report, Vol. 31 (Sept. 24, 1982), pp. 507–514.

focuses exclusively on the severe, late signs and symptoms of infection with the virus.

The following pages examine the incidence and characteristics of some of the more common signs of AIDS and then describe other conditions known to be caused by HTLV-III/LAV. The latter include an acute mononucleosis-like disease that may appear shortly after infection with the virus; lymphadenopathy syndrome and AIDS-related complex; non-Hodgkin's lymphomas; and HTLV-III/LAV infection of the brain. The final section outlines some of the differences between AIDS in adults and in children.

Opportunistic Infections

HTLV-III/LAV destroys the body's defensive capabilities, opening the door to any disease-producing agents present in the environment. In populations that have a high incidence of tuberculosis—such as intravenous drug abusers and immigrants from some developing countries—AIDS is associated with extremely aggressive tubercular lesions in sites not usually affected by the bacterium. Africans with AIDS are prone to cryptococcal meningitis, an infection caused by a yeastlike organism. The parasitic disease toxoplasmosis occurs frequently among AIDS patients born in Haiti. Homosexuals with AIDS often develop persistent herpes infections because the immune cells that had kept the virus in check are destroyed.

Pneumocystis carinii Pneumonia

The most common life-threatening opportunistic infection in AIDS patients is *Pneumocystis carinii* pneumonia, a parasitic infection previously seen almost exclusively in cancer and transplant patients receiving immunosuppressive drugs. The first signs of this disorder are moderate to severe difficulty in breathing, dry cough, and fever.

P. carinii pneumonia occurs at least once in more than two-thirds of all AIDS patients. An analysis by the New York

Department of Health found that the average survival time for patients whose diagnosis of AIDS was based on *P. carinii* pneumonia alone was 35 weeks.

With early diagnosis and appropriate drug therapy, about 90 percent of AIDS patients survive their first episode of this disease, but most require longer treatment than transplant or cancer patients with the same symptoms. In one study, almost 75 percent of AIDS patients continued to have high concentrations of *P. carinii* in their lungs after two to three weeks of therapy. In contrast, most other patients treated for this infection have no detectable parasites within 3 to 14 days after treatment begins.

Another problem in treating AIDS patients with *P. carinii* pneumonia is that an unexpectedly large number have adverse reactions to sulfa drugs. The reasons for this phenomenon are unknown, although a similar intolerance has been reported in patients with other immune-system defects.

About a fifth of AIDS patients who respond to therapy for *P. carinii* pneumonia relapse, and those who do not eventually succumb to another infection. Efforts are under way to develop new and better drug regimens to fight these infections, but long-term survival of future AIDS patients probably will depend on specific therapies to block the effects of HTLV-III/LAV.

Cytomegalovirus

The majority of patients with AIDS have active cytomegalovirus (CMV) infections. This virus is a member of the herpesvirus group. The most common sign of its presence in AIDS patients is spots on the retina, which may lead to blindness. The virus also causes pneumonia, esophagitis, and colitis. CMV infection may be the principal cause of death in some cases. Many researchers believe that CMV infection may be linked to the development of Kaposi's sarcoma, but this relationship has not been proved.

CMV infection rarely produces clinical symptoms in healthy adults, although it does cause some cases of a mononucleosis-like syndrome. Before the appearance of AIDS, the populations most at risk from CMV were newborns with congenital infections and transplant and cancer patients receiving immunosuppressive drugs.

CMV infections generally respond poorly to antiviral chemotherapy, but several new drugs have shown promise in clinical trials. Among AIDS patients, however, clinical improvements have been brief and relapses common. Control of CMV infections in these patients probably will require the development of new medications that are suitable for long-term therapy.

Candida albicans

Infection with *Candida albicans*, a yeastlike fungus, may be one of the first signs of an immune system weakened by HTLV-III/LAV. In patients with AIDS-related complex, the whitish mouth sores characteristic of candidiasis (commonly called thrush) indicate a high risk of developing AIDS. AIDS patients often have candidiasis lesions that extend into the esophagus, and a few patients have been reported with candidiasis lesions in the brain.

Infections with *C. albicans* usually respond to antifungal therapy, but in patients with AIDS the disease often reappears as soon as therapy has been completed.

Toxoplasma gondii

The protozoan parasite *Toxoplasma gondii* is one of the most common causes of encephalitis (inflammation of the brain) in patients with AIDS. Most patients improve clinically within two to three weeks of the start of appropriate therapy, but relapses are common even after six months of treatment. Patients who appear to recover need careful follow-up; many medical centers continue therapy indefinitely.

Mycobacterium avium-intracellulare

Almost one-third of AIDS patients treated at the National Institutes of Health have had *Mycobacterium avium-intracellulare* infections in the brain or other locations outside the lung. This bacterium, related to the organism that causes tuberculosis in humans, was rarely seen by physicians before the appearance of AIDS. It is extremely difficult to treat, in part because most strains are resistant to conventional antibiotics.

Cryptosporidium

The protozoan parasite *Cryptosporidium* causes severe, protracted diarrhea. Scientists have been interested in the organism for many years because of its effect on calves and other domestic animals. The first recognized case of human cryptosporidiosis occurred in 1976.

In persons with a normal immune system, *Cryptosporidium* causes a self-limited disease that lasts one to two weeks. In AIDS patients the diarrhea often becomes chronic and may lead to severe malnutrition. Treatment of this disorder remains experimental, but several drugs have shown promise in some patients.

Tuberculosis

Tuberculosis is not usually considered an opportunistic infection, but there is new evidence that the AIDS epidemic may be causing a resurgence of the disease in the United States. This finding is of special concern, because tuberculosis is more contagious than most infections that take advantage of the weakened immune system in AIDS. It has the potential to spread beyond AIDS patients into the general population. Tuberculosis in AIDS patients usually responds to therapy.

The preceding descriptions illustrate the diagnostic and treatment challenges presented by AIDS-related infections. Some of these infections were extremely rare before 1981 and are still unfamiliar to the majority of practicing physicians. Others are well known but consistently resist even the most advanced therapeutic techniques. The potential impact of a large patient population with multiple infections of this type is difficult to imagine. It underscores the importance of developing new techniques to rebuild dismantled immune systems and to block the primary culprit, HTLV-III/LAV.

Kaposi's Sarcoma

The signs of Kaposi's sarcoma are blue-violet to brownish skin blotches or bumps. When the first blotch appears it may be mistaken for a bruise; but unlike a bruise it does not go away after a week or 10 days. Kaposi's sarcoma is a cancer or tumor of the blood vessel walls. Before the appearance of AIDS it was rare in the United States and Europe, where it occurred primarily in men over 55 or 60, usually of Mediterranean origin.

More than 93 percent of AIDS patients who have Kaposi's sarcoma are homosexual or bisexual men. For those in whom Kaposi's sarcoma is the first sign of AIDS, the average survival time is slightly more than two and a half years. Studies of the immune systems of these patients indicate that they generally are less depleted than those of patients whose AIDS diagnosis is based on an opportunistic infection.

Kaposi's sarcoma is rarely life threatening for the middle-aged and elderly men who develop the disease in the absence of AIDS. Their lesions usually occur on the legs, grow very slowly, and do not invade other tissues. But the epidemic form of the disease is quite different. More than 75 percent of AIDS patients with Kaposi's sarcoma have disseminated disease, usually involving the lymph nodes, the lungs, or the gastrointestinal tract. Physicians treating AIDS patients in San Francisco have found several cases of Kaposi's sarcoma in the brain, a phenomenon that had been reported only once before in the scientific literature.

Many different therapeutic approaches have been employed to treat AIDS-related Kaposi's sarcoma. Between 30 and 40 percent of patients respond initially to alpha interferon, a natural substance that stimulates the immune cells most affected by HTLV-III/LAV. Radiation therapy sometimes produces temporary reductions in superficial lesions, and aggressive chemotherapy in the late stages of disease may produce sufficient improvement to allow a hospitalized patient to return home. Kaposi's sarcoma rarely is the principal cause of death in these patients, but it may be extremely debilitating and it further weakens patients who eventually succumb to opportunistic infections.

Three aspects of Kaposi's sarcoma in AIDS have puzzled scientists: its tendency to behave like an opportunistic infection; its predominance in homosexual men; and the gradual decline in the proportion of AIDS patients with this form of cancer.

Answers to the first two puzzles may be related in part to the apparent connection between Kaposi's sarcoma and CMV. Researchers in central Africa, where classic Kaposi's sarcoma is more prevalent than in the United States, have found several types of evidence linking this virus to cancer. For example, in tissue samples from patients with Kaposi's sarcoma, cancer cells appear to carry the genetic blueprint for CMV while surrounding normal cells do not. In addition, laboratory studies have shown that CMV can trigger unregulated, cancerous growth in hamster cells.

Blood samples from homosexual men indicate that more than 90 percent have been exposed to CMV, a much higher proportion than among other groups at risk of AIDS. In some of these men the virus probably establishes a latent infection—it hides in a few cells until a breach in the body's defense mechanisms allows it to reemerge. The immune defects produced by HTLV-III/LAV appear to be sufficient to trigger this reactivation.

Other studies suggest that some people may have an inherited tendency to develop Kaposi's sarcoma. Researchers have discovered characteristic markers on blood cells from patients with both classic and AIDS-associated forms of this cancer. Perhaps CMV can trigger Kaposi's sarcoma only in those with a genetic susceptibility to the disease.

No explanation is available for the recent decline in the proportion of AIDS patients with Kaposi's sarcoma. Before 1984 Kaposi's sarcoma accounted for 21 percent of reported

AIDS diagnoses; between January 1985 and December 1985 it accounted for only 13 percent of diagnoses.

Acute Infection with HTLV-III/LAV

Physicians monitoring the health of almost 1,000 homosexual and bisexual men in Sydney, Australia, discovered that a mononucleosis-like disease sometimes develops shortly after infection with HTLV-III/LAV. The disease lasts from 3 to 14 days and is associated with fevers, sweats, exhaustion, loss of appetite, nausea, headaches, sore throat, diarrhea, swollen glands, and a rash on the trunk.

In one patient in the Australian study, the illness developed 6 days after probable exposure. Three other patients developed antibodies against the virus 19, 32, and 56 days after onset of the illness. Laboratory studies showed that all of the patients had some immunologic abnormalities, but not the extreme changes seen in AIDS patients.

The significance of this acute illness in terms of the future health of affected patients is not known. Physicians will watch closely to determine if there is a relationship between the initial response to HTLV-III/LAV infection and the subsequent development of AIDS or other problems. (As noted earlier, the interval between infection and diagnosis of AIDS may be quite long. The average incubation period for transfusion-associated AIDS is about four and a half years. Among homosexual men who develop AIDS, the average interval between the appearance of HTLV-III/LAV antibodies and diagnosis of full-blown disease is more than three years.)

Lymphadenopathy Syndrome and the AIDS-Related Complex

Soon after AIDS was identified as a new syndrome, physicians began to notice that a much larger group of previously healthy homosexual men was seeking treatment for persistent swollen glands not explained by specific illnesses or drug use. The epidemiologic characteristics (age, racial composition, and residential patterns) of this population were identical to those of the population of AIDS patients. As the epidemic progressed, similar findings were reported among intravenous drug abusers, hemophiliacs, and the heterosexual partners of some AIDS patients.

The presence of multiple swollen glands for more than three months without other signs of disease was labeled chronic lymphadenopathy syndrome. Often, however, the lymphadenopathy was just one element among a constellation of ongoing problems, including unintentional weight loss, fever, diarrhea, lethargy, a variety of immunologic abnormalities (similar to but usually less severe than those appearing in AIDS patients), and oral thrush (*C. albicans* infection). Gradually, most physicians adopted the umbrella term "AIDS-related complex" to encompass all these abnormalities.

When the blood test for HTLV-III/LAV antibodies became available, researchers demonstrated that more than a quarter of those infected with the virus developed lymphadenopathy or laboratory evidence of related conditions. Early studies showed that between 6 and 20 percent of these patients eventually developed the full-blown syndrome. For example, a San Francisco study found a 7 percent incidence of AIDS among lymphadenopathy patients after 36 months.

More recent data suggest that the frequency of progression from ARC to AIDS may be higher, at least in some populations. Among one group of homosexual men with generalized lymphadenopathy followed by researchers at Mount Sinai School of Medicine in New York City, 8 of 42 patients (19 percent) converted to AIDS within 30 months, and 12 of 42 patients (29 percent) converted within $4\frac{1}{2}$ years. Two explanations could account for the variation between the New York and San Francisco studies: the New York patients may have been infected with the virus HTLV-III/LAV longer (the epidemic is believed to have started in New York about a year before it appeared in California), or they may have had a higher incidence of certain "cofactors" that increase the risk of disease. (Chapter 6 describes the search for potential cofactors.)

Despite these figures, ARC should not automatically be

considered a form of "pre-AIDS." The majority of patients with chronic lymphadenopathy syndrome or ARC remain stable, at least for five years (clinical experience with HTLV-III/LAV infections is still relatively brief), and some appear to improve. ARC patients who require medical care early in their clinical course seem to be at greatest risk. In 1984 the Mount Sinai researchers and their co-workers reported that conversion from chronic lymphadenopathy syndrome to AIDS was associated with previous heavy use of recreational drugs (nitrite inhalants); night sweats; decreased white blood cell counts; and the combination of clinical symptoms, low white cell count, and enlarged spleen.

The impact of ARC on a patient's life-style varies tremendously, depending on the symptoms. Most ARC patients continue working and have long periods of relative comfort, but for some, the diarrhea and fevers may be as debilitating as AIDS itself. These men and women may be bedridden and often require extensive supportive services.

Lymphomas and HTLV-III/LAV Infection

Between 1980 and 1983, cancer registry data in the San Francisco Bay Area and in Los Angeles County showed a threefold increase in the number of young, never-married men with high-grade lymphomas, which are aggressive cancers characterized by unregulated proliferation of certain white blood cells. Most of the affected men were homosexuals; many had generalized lymphadenopathy when their cancers were diagnosed, and some had AIDS.

Clinical researchers now believe that non-Hodgkin's lymphomas in patients at high risk of AIDS are another sign of infection with HTLV-III/LAV. These lymphomas resemble cancers that develop in children with congenital immune defects. The tumors often appear outside the lymph nodes, and most respond poorly to treatment.

In one study of 90 homosexual lymphoma patients from four major cities, 42 percent were diagnosed with tumors in the central nervous system (23 percent directly in the brain), and 33 percent had bone marrow involvement. (The frequency of lymphoma of the brain in other patients with similar types of lymphoma is about 2 percent.) Kaposi's sarcoma or severe opportunistic infections characteristic of AIDS developed in almost half of those who had generalized lymphadenopathy at diagnosis and in 3 of 12 who initially had no AIDS-related conditions. Patients who had evidence of ARC or AIDS were less likely to respond to treatment, relapsed more frequently, and had a higher mortality rate.

These findings indicate that lymphoma may precede AIDS in some patients. Several different theories have been proposed to explain why. HTLV-III/LAV does not appear to cause cancer on its own, but it may depress immune functions sufficiently to allow other viruses to act. For example, many homosexual men have evidence of exposure to the herpesvirus Epstein–Barr virus (EBV). EBV has been implicated as a causal factor in the development of Burkitt's lymphoma in Africa (Burkitt's lymphoma is very difficult to distinguish microscopically from the lymphomas most common in AIDS patients) and of nasopharyngeal carcinoma in susceptible persons in the Far East. Abnormalities of immune regulation caused by infection with HTLV-III/LAV may allow EBV to initiate the processes that eventually lead to cancer.

Non-Hodgkin's lymphoma is included in the case definition of AIDS only if it is limited to the brain or if it occurs in association with a positive test for HTLV-III/LAV (see Appendix A). Other cases are not included because lymphomas may cause, as well as result from, damage to the immune system.

HTLV-III/LAV Infection in the Brain

About one-third of patients with AIDS develop a degenerative brain disorder caused directly by HTLV-III/LAV infection of brain cells. In adults, the disorder usually begins with diminished concentration and mild memory loss and progresses to severe mental deterioration (see Figure 7). Some patients also develop numbness in the limbs that may lead to paralysis.

Signs of brain degeneration in infants and young children

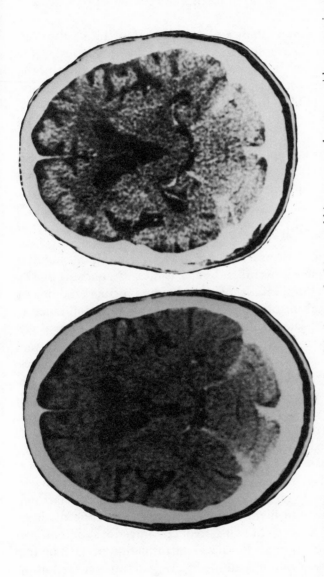

FIGURE 7. Computerized axial tomography of the brain of a 36-year-old intravenous drug user with progressive memory loss and other signs of AIDS. *Left:* Three months after onset he had moderate dementia—scan shows atrophy of the cortex, or surface, of the brain and enlargement of the ventricles (spaces within the brain). *Right:* Six months after onset he had severe dementia—scan shows further dilation of the ventricles and progressive atrophy of both the cortex and the white matter of the brain. Source: Reprinted, with permission, from Richard T. Johnson and Justin C. McArthur, "AIDS and the Brain," *Trends in Neuroscience,* Vol. 9, No. 3 (March 1986), pp. 91–94.

may include the loss of developmental milestones (for example, a baby who had been able to sit or to talk becomes unable to do so), seizures, and the absence of age-appropriate growth of the head.

Recent reports indicate that HTLV-III/LAV also can cause acute and chronic meningitis, and may be responsible for degeneration of the spinal cord and abnormalities of the peripheral nervous system in some AIDS and ARC patients. Moreover, HTLV-III/LAV-related neurologic disease may occur before or in the absence of immune-system defects. The prospect of large numbers of patients with AIDS-related mental disorders underscores the need for a drug that can suppress the effects of this virus in the brain as well as in the bloodstream and other tissues.

AIDS in Children

Pediatric AIDS is a different disease from AIDS in adults, especially when it occurs in young babies. Diagnosing AIDS in the very young can be difficult, because infants tend not to get the opportunistic infections and cancers common in adult patients until late in the course of their illnesses; yet early diagnosis is essential because of their extreme vulnerability.

Another factor that complicates the identification of pediatric AIDS is that initial clinical signs often resemble those associated with inherited defects of the immune system. Common symptoms include failure to thrive (weight loss), chronic diarrhea, and frequent bacterial infections.

As noted earlier, those at risk of pediatric AIDS include infants born into families in which one or both parents have AIDS or are at high risk of developing AIDS, children who received blood transfusions from subjects with risk factors, and children with hemophilia. The presence of one of these risk factors in a child with frequent infections or chronic interstitial pneumonitis (localized inflammation of the lung for more than two months) immediately leads to a suspicion of AIDS, but confirmation of the diagnosis depends on appropriate laboratory tests.

The most common immunologic finding in children with AIDS is an extremely high level of antibodies in the blood. Paradoxically, the cells that make these antibodies are unable to respond appropriately when challenged with a substance that normally elicits an immune response. Changes in other measures of immune function usually occur as the disease progresses. The blood test for HTLV-III/LAV antibodies has proved to be a tremendous asset in distinguishing AIDS from other immunodeficiency diseases, but it may not be conclusive in young babies (who may still have antibodies acquired from their mothers before birth). In infants under six months of age, a diagnosis of HTLV-III/LAV infection should be based on isolation of the virus from blood samples.

One of the most worrisome aspects of immune deficiency in children with AIDS is the theoretical possibility that the young patients will be unable to tolerate vaccines. Some of today's vaccines, including those against polio and measles, contain live viruses. These viruses have been altered in the laboratory so that they elicit a protective response without causing disease; but the AIDS patient may not be strong enough to withstand even these weakened microbes. At least one case has been reported of an adult with unrecognized AIDS who developed a severe adverse reaction following immunization with smallpox vaccine. In populations with a high prevalence of HTLV-III/LAV infection (such as those in central Africa), the inability to tolerate vaccines could become an extremely serious public health problem.

Conclusion

AIDS—defined as the presence of a disease indicative of immune deficiency in a patient with no known cause of diminished resistance to that disease—is only one of the manifestations of infection with HTLV-III/LAV. The majority of those infected remain free of clinical symptoms for at least the first two to five years, although they can transmit the virus to others through sexual contact or through an exchange of blood or blood products. About one-fourth of those infected develop lymphadenopathy syndrome or another AIDS-related condition. Most patients with lymphadenopathy alone have remained stable for the periods studied, and some have improved.

A much smaller group of patients infected with HTLV-III/LAV develop a cancer not included in the original definition of AIDS, such as non-Hodgkin's lymphoma. Tumors in these patients often occur at sites, such as the brain, not usually affected by primary lymphomas in other populations. Cancer patients who have ARC or AIDS at diagnosis or who develop AIDS during cancer therapy have higher recurrence and mortality rates than other patients.

Pediatric AIDS is more difficult to diagnose than adult AIDS, in part because of possible confusion with inherited defects of the immune system. Also, infants often lack the familiar clinical and laboratory signs of AIDS. They are more likely to succumb to bacterial diseases than to the spectrum of opportunistic infections seen in older patients. Techniques to isolate HTLV-III/LAV from blood samples and licensed antibody tests now make it possible to identify these children early; thus they can receive the medical and social support they need.

Both adult and pediatric AIDS patients may show signs of AIDS encephalopathy, a degenerative brain disease. Recent reports indicate that this and other HTLV-III/LAV-related neurologic conditions can occur in patients who have no other clinical symptoms of AIDS. Researchers expect a considerable increase in these neurologic complications as the incidence of infection rises in the United States.

* * *

Chapter 3 is based on the presentations of Anthony S. Fauci, National Institute of Allergy and Infectious Diseases; Robert C. Gallo, National Cancer Institute; James W. Curran, Centers for Disease Control; Richard T. Johnson, Johns Hopkins University School of Medicine; and Luc Montagnier, Institut Pasteur. The case histories described at the beginning of the chapter are based on articles in the *Journal of the American Medical Association*, June 21, 1985, pp. 3425–3428, 3428–3430.

4

Discovery of the Virus

The battle against AIDS illustrates both the power and the limitations of recent advances in molecular biology, virology, and recombinant DNA technology. Less than five years after the disease first attracted attention, researchers had identified the virus that causes it, deciphered its genetic code, and developed a versatile and inexpensive screening test. Yet these monumental achievements do not mean that there will be a rapid solution to the AIDS problem. The screening test will help control the spread of infection, but eradication of the disease will be a long and difficult process.

This chapter sketches the search for and the discovery of the virus now called HTLV-III/LAV, its relationship to other disease-producing microorganisms, and its possible origin in central Africa. It also examines the characteristics of the virus that complicate development of an AIDS vaccine and of specific short-term therapies.

Understanding the Problem

When the first cases of *Pneumocystis carinii* pneumonia and Kaposi's sarcoma were reported in young, previously healthy homosexual men in the spring of 1981, speculation began immediately about possible causes. What had changed these men from active members of the community to seriously ill invalids in just a few months?

Physicians immediately focused on the immune systems

of the first AIDS patients. In December 1981 the *New England Journal of Medicine* carried three articles describing immunologic evaluations of 19 homosexual patients with *P. carinii* pneumonia or an unusually persistent herpes infection. All of the 19 men had reduced numbers of T lymphocytes, white blood cells that play a key role in protecting the body against disease. Subsequent studies showed that one particular subset of T lymphocytes, consisting of cells carrying a T4 surface marker, was dramatically reduced in AIDS.

As the epidemic spread through major urban homosexual communities in the United States, theories about the cause of the syndrome multiplied. The possibility of an unknown infectious agent was considered, but early laboratory studies failed to identify a suspect. The life-styles of individual patients were compared with those of healthy homosexuals to highlight any differences that might explain susceptibility to the disease.

Interviews with patients indicated that they tended to be more sexually active than matched populations of healthy homosexuals. Researchers speculated that repeated infections acquired during hundreds of sexual encounters might have overwhelmed the T lymphocytes in these patients, leaving them unable to fight disease. Another theory rested on the immunosuppressive properties of human semen, which could have entered the bloodstream through small tears in the rectum during anal intercourse.

Illicit drug use also was viewed as a potential cause. In February 1982 James J. Goedert and his colleagues at the National Institutes of Health and the Uniformed Services University of the Health Sciences described immunologic defects associated with the use of amyl nitrite, a drug sometimes used by homosexuals as a sexual stimulant. They speculated that nitrites might be immunosuppressive in the presence of repeated viral infections (laboratory studies later demonstrated that nitrites are not immunosuppressive).

The focus on life-styles continued during the first quarter of 1982, when the disease began appearing in heterosexual men and women who were intravenous drug abusers. This population appeared to have many of the same risk factors as promiscuous homosexuals. The practice of needle sharing caused a high incidence of multiple infections, and some of the most commonly abused drugs were known to be immunosuppressants.

Epidemiologists at the Centers for Disease Control in Atlanta continued to maintain close surveillance of new cases. They documented clusters of disease both in homosexual men and among IV drug abusers. These clusters were analogous to those produced by the spread of hepatitis B infection in high-risk populations. Their presence supported the theory that AIDS was transmitted by an infectious microorganism.

This theory achieved even greater prominence in July 1982 when, as described in Chapter 2, three cases of AIDS were reported in hemophiliacs who had been treated with clotting-factor concentrates to prevent bleeding. Further evidence for the existence of a specific agent transmitted by both sexual contact and blood products accumulated in late 1982 and early 1983.

Laboratories in the United States and in Europe rallied to the search for the AIDS agent. Some investigators believed that the syndrome might represent a new manifestation of a known virus; both cytomegalovirus and Epstein-Barr virus had been shown to suppress the immune system, but neither seemed capable of causing the kind of devastation associated with AIDS. Others suspected that the disease might be caused by a co-infection with two or more microorganisms. Finally, research teams began searching for an entirely new viral pathogen.

The urgency of the problem and the growing public concern over it were reflected in frequent newspaper headlines about AIDS. Existing therapies could not stop the progression of the disease, and the number of reported cases was increasing geometrically.

Suspicion Falls on the Retroviruses

The idea that a retrovirus might be involved in AIDS crystallized in early 1982 as a result of discussions between Robert C. Gallo of the National Cancer Institute (NCI) and

Myron Essex of the Harvard School of Public Health. The first human retrovirus had been isolated only four years earlier by Gallo and his colleagues in the NCI Laboratory of Tumor Cell Biology; until publication of their report on this work, many scientists had believed that retroviruses might not cause human disease.

The basic structure of the retrovirus is similar to that of other viruses: it consists of a tightly packed core of genetic material wrapped in a protective protein sheath. The molecule carrying the genetic information in the retrovirus is RNA (ribonucleic acid).

In living cells, RNA functions as a messenger between the cell nucleus, which contains the more familiar genetic material DNA (deoxyribonucleic acid), and the rest of the cell. When a new protein is needed for a particular function or structure, the portion of the DNA molecule coding for that protein is transcribed into RNA. The RNA molecule then migrates out of the nucleus into the cytoplasm, where it directs the manufacture of the new protein.

The unique feature of the retrovirus is that it reverses this process. Each virus particle carries the enzyme reverse transcriptase, which copies the single-stranded viral RNA into double-stranded DNA (see Figure 8). The viral DNA migrates into the cell nucleus, where it forms a circle and then inserts itself into the host cell DNA. The integrated viral DNA is called a provirus. If the host cell divides, a copy of the provirus is transmitted to each daughter cell. In addition, the viral DNA can co-opt the genetic machinery of its host to produce large quantities of viral RNA, some of which is packaged into new virus particles and released by budding through the cell membrane (see Figure 9).

The American pathologist Francis Peyton Rous was the first person to isolate a retrovirus, in 1911. He identified it as the cause of a particular type of cancer, known as a sarcoma, in chickens. The Rous sarcoma virus is a member of the subfamily Oncovirinae. Other members of this group cause leukemias and lymphomas in cats, mice, and cows. For the past 20 years, most research on retroviruses has focused on the

LIFE CYCLE OF A RETROVIRUS

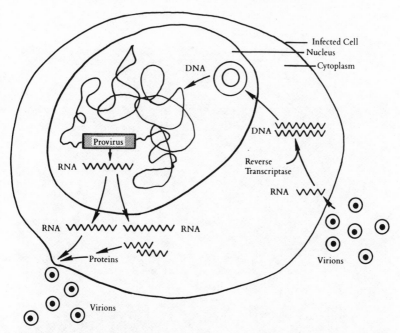

FIGURE 8.   During the life cycle of a retrovirus, intact virus particles (virions) are taken into the cell via a specific cellular receptor. After uncoating, the single-stranded RNA is transcribed into double-stranded DNA. The DNA enters the cell nucleus where it forms a circle and integrates itself into the host cell genome. The integrated viral DNA is called a provirus. In some cases the provirus remains dormant or unexpressed. In other cases it is transcribed into viral RNA, leading to the production of viral proteins and the formation of new virus particles. These progeny virions are released by budding from the cell membrane. Courtesy of Robert C. Gallo, Laboratory of Tumor Cell Biology, National Cancer Institute.

oncoviruses. There has been less emphasis on a second subfamily, Lentivirinae. Until recently, the only known lentiviruses caused encephalitis, anemia, pneumonia, or arthritis in sheep, goats, and horses.

The first human retrovirus, isolated by Gallo and colleagues in 1978, was from the cells of an American man with

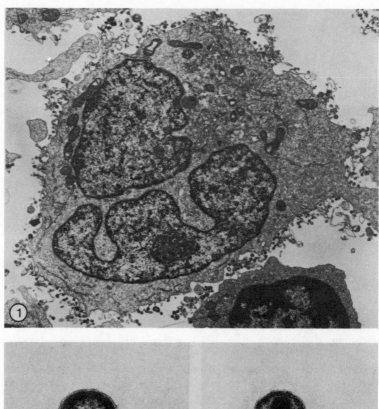

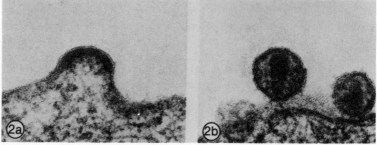

FIGURE 9. Electronmicrographs of (1) HTLV-III/LAV-infected cell (×15,000) and (2a, 2b) budding of virus from the cell membrane (×90,000). Courtesy of Syed Zaki Salahuddin, National Cancer Institute.

T-cell leukemia. In published reports of the finding in 1980, Gallo and his co-workers labeled this retrovirus "human T-cell leukemia/lymphoma virus" (HTLV). Additional studies demonstrated that the T4 helper cell was the principal target of this new virus.

Several years later, Japanese and American scientists demonstrated that HTLV was the cause of adult T-cell leukemia syndrome (ATL), an endemic disease in certain parts of southwestern Japan. Further studies uncovered many other endemic areas, including Caribbean islands, the southeastern United States, areas in South America and in southern Italy, and many parts of Africa. Meanwhile, a second but much rarer HTLV virus (HTLV-II) was isolated from the cells of another American leukemia patient.

The discovery of a virus very similar to HTLV-I—simian T-lymphotropic virus type I, or STLV-I—in African green monkeys and several other primate species provided an important clue to the ancestry of the human virus. Many researchers believe that HTLV-I originated in Africa, where a progenitor made the transition from monkeys to humans. Gallo speculates that this new human pathogen was carried to other continents by European commercial and slave traders who traveled the shipping routes between Africa, Asia, and the Americas beginning in about the sixteenth century.

Isolating the AIDS Virus

Several facts supported the theory that a human retrovirus caused AIDS:

1. Some animal retroviruses (including feline leukemia virus) were known to cause an AIDS-like disease as well as cancer.
2. Like HTLV-I and HTLV-II, the AIDS agent seemed to disrupt the function of T4 cells.
3. The suspected modes of transmission of AIDS, through blood products and sexual contact, appeared identical to those implicated in the transmission of HTLV-I. (Leuke-

mias caused by HTLV-I infection are very rare in the United States; there is no evidence that other forms of leukemia are transmitted by sexual contact or transfusions.)

4. Patients with adult T-cell leukemia also were subject to numerous opportunistic infections, and T cells infected with HTLV-I and HTLV-II showed suppressed immune activity in the laboratory.

5. Although AIDS was first recognized in the United States, a growing number of cases from Haiti and reports of a similar disease in Africa suggested an origin similar to that proposed for HTLV-I.

Even with this knowledge, efforts to isolate the AIDS agent proved to be extremely frustrating. Scientists occasionally could detect transient reverse transcriptase activity in cultured T cells from patients with AIDS or related conditions, but the results were not reproducible. The major problem was that researchers could not maintain the virus or the T cells in culture. Only later did they learn that the virus was killing the cells before they could complete their analyses.

The first isolation of the virus later shown to be the cause of AIDS was reported in May 1983 by Luc Montagnier, head of the Viral Oncology Unit of the Pasteur Institute in Paris, and his colleagues. They named the virus lymphadenopathy-associated virus (LAV), because they had isolated it from one of the swollen lymph nodes of a patient with lymphadenopathy syndrome (these patients appeared to be at high risk of developing AIDS). Over the next few months, similar retroviruses were isolated by the Pasteur group from the blood of several AIDS patients, but the researchers continued to have problems with virus propagation.

In May 1984 Mikulas Popovic and his co-workers in Gallo's laboratory reported in the journal *Science* that they had identified a line of cancerous T cells that had two important characteristics: (1) susceptibility to infection with the new virus and (2) the ability to resist the killing effects that had destroyed other infected T-cell cultures. In fact, cultures of this cell line could be adapted to produce large quantities of the virus for research and for the development of a much-needed screening test.

The NCI researchers reported that they had isolated the new virus, which they designated HTLV-III, from 48 patients. The meaning of HTLV was changed from "human T-cell leukemia/lymphoma virus" to "human T-cell lymphotropic virus" to reflect the fact that all members of the HTLV family shared an attraction to T lymphocytes.

Another virus isolate was described in August 1984 by Jay Levy and his co-workers from the University of California at San Francisco. They named their virus AIDS-associated retrovirus, or ARV.

Molecular analysis of isolates from many different AIDS and ARC patients (researchers determined the identity and position of each nucleotide or chemical building block in the viral RNA genome) demonstrated that they were all variants of the same virus. Most of the scientific community applauded this discovery—a known enemy is easier to fight—but controversy abounded about the name of the virus, as is discussed later in this chapter. In the United States most scientific journals have used the designation HTLV-III/LAV.*

Much additional work was required to prove that HTLV-III/LAV actually causes AIDS and that it is not simply another opportunistic infection attacking a host that is defenseless for some other reason. Between mid-1983 and late 1984, researchers on both sides of the Atlantic searched for signs of HTLV-III/LAV infection in the blood of hundreds of healthy volunteers from low-risk groups, genetically immunodeficient patients, healthy individuals from high-risk groups, patients with lymphadenopathy syndrome (persistent swollen glands), and AIDS patients. These studies consistently demonstrated that the acquisition and transmission of HTLV-III/LAV correlated with AIDS or AIDS-related conditions.

Blood recipients who developed AIDS and their high-risk

---

*A proposal for a consensus name for the virus is under study by the Retrovirus Study Group of the International Committee on the Taxonomy of Viruses.

donors provided an extremely important piece of the puzzle. The detailed records kept by blood banks allowed the researchers to trace the natural history of the disease as it was transmitted from one individual to another. Identical virus isolates could be obtained from blood recipients with AIDS (with no other source of infection) and from the high-risk donors who gave the blood.

The Diversity of the Virus

Subsequent analysis of different HTLV-III/LAV isolates produced one very disturbing finding. Although the isolates were unquestionably representatives of the same virus, they differed by a surprising amount. For example, more than 6 percent of the genetic building blocks in ARV were different from those in early HTLV-III isolates (which came from patients in New York City); other pairs of isolates differed by even greater amounts. This variation suggested an unusually high rate of spontaneous change—mutation—in the genetic material.

Further analysis has revealed that most of the nucleotide differences among HTLV-III/LAV viruses occur in the portion of the viral RNA coding for the envelope protein. As explained below, this may hamper efforts to develop an AIDS vaccine.

The envelope is the protective coat that shields the core of the virus from the environment (see Figure 10). Because it is on the outside, it is also the most likely part of the virus to elicit a response from the immune system. One facet of this response is the production of antibody molecules that recognize and bind to specific portions of the envelope protein. Antibody binding then triggers other immune processes that lead to destruction of the virus (antibodies also may be made against other components of the virus, but these are rarely protective).

Conventional vaccines use a killed whole virus or a live attentuated virus (a virus particle tamed in the laboratory to prevent it from causing disease) to elicit the same protective antibodies that would be produced during natural infection.

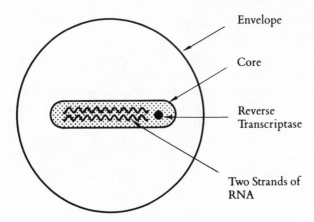

Envelope

Core

Reverse
Transcriptase

Two Strands of
RNA

FIGURE 10. Schematic diagram of HTLV-III/LAV. Source: Adapted, with permission, from "Why the AIDS Virus Is Not Like HTLVs-I or -II," *New Scientist*, Vol. 105, No. 1442 (Feb. 7, 1985), p. 4.

New subunit vaccines employ a molecule similar or identical to a piece of the viral protein coat to accomplish the same task.

The problem with a virus that changes its coat rapidly is that antibodies made against the envelope protein of one viral isolate may not be protective against another isolate. The impact of the genetic variation among HTLV-III/LAV isolates on vaccine prospects will not be known definitely until researchers learn more about the structure of the envelope protein and its interaction with neutralizing antibodies.

Several factors could explain the high mutation rate of HTLV-III/LAV. One possibility is that its reverse transcriptase molecule may be less accurate than enzymes that regulate DNA synthesis in other systems—it may be more likely to substitute one chemical building block for another.

Explosive Replication

Another factor that makes HTLV-III/LAV a particularly formidable opponent is the pace at which new virus particles are produced. William Haseltine of the Dana-Farber Cancer Institute in Boston and his co-workers were the first to describe the startling replication rate of HTLV-III/LAV. Like

HTLV-I and HTLV-II and certain other animal viruses, HTLV-III/LAV has a mechanism that allows it to control the speed at which viral genes are expressed (transcribed into RNA and then translated into proteins).

The Boston researchers, in collaboration with NCI investigators in Gallo's laboratory, have pinpointed the viral gene responsible for this activity in HTLV-III/LAV—they call it the *trans*-activator or *tat*-III gene—and have made major strides in understanding its effects. Their most significant finding is that HTLV-III/LAV has a different mechanism of *trans*-activation from that of HTLV-I and HTLV-II. The increase in gene expression in HTLV-I and HTLV-II results from an increase in the rate at which viral DNA is transcribed into RNA. In contrast, the protein product of the *tat*-III gene regulates post-transcriptional events; it increases the efficiency of RNA translation into viral proteins.

Another important discovery, reported independently by Dana-Farber and NCI scientists in March 1986, is that the protein product of the *tat*-III gene is essential for viral replication. Using techniques of genetic engineering, the researchers deleted the *tat*-III gene from HTLV-III/LAV proviruses. They expected that a virus without a *tat*-III gene would replicate much more slowly than a normal virus—instead they found that it could not replicate at all. T-cell cultures exposed to the defective virus remained healthy.

These findings have important implications for the development of new antiviral drugs. Efforts are under way to identify drugs that can inhibit the *tat*-III gene without disrupting the function of human cells.

The Link Between HTLV-III/LAV and the Lentiviruses

The unexpected swiftness of HTLV-III/LAV gene expression and the extent of variation among HTLV-III/LAV isolates set this virus apart from other members of the HTLV family. In addition, the HTLV-III/LAV provirus can function outside the nucleus; it does not have to integrate into the host cell DNA to replicate.

These factors, combined with the different biological effects of the viruses (HTLV-I and HTLV-II cause T-cell proliferation, but HTLV-III causes cell death), have led some researchers to suggest that HTLV-III is an inappropriate name for the virus that causes AIDS. Gallo and others disagree, citing the facts that all three viruses exhibit a strong preference for the T4 cell, that they have identical modes of transmission, and that portions of their RNA genomes are similar.

Whatever their positions on the name issue, however, most researchers agree that HTLV-I and HTLV-II occupy one branch of the retrovirus family tree, and HTLV-III/LAV another. The first two share many features with animal oncoviruses (such as bovine leukemia virus), while the structure and function of HTLV-III/LAV place it firmly in the subfamily Lentivirinae. The importance of this relationship is that knowledge about the animal lentiviruses may provide clues about disease patterns and preventive approaches to AIDS.

When the lentiviruses infect domestic sheep, goats, and horses, one hallmark of the resulting diseases is progressive neurological impairment caused by the gradual death of brain cells. Recent evidence indicates that HTLV-III/LAV also may replicate in brain cells and may destroy them. The first clinical signs of this process in humans may be impaired concentration or memory loss; some patients eventually progress to severe dementia. HTLV-III/LAV-related neurological disease may occur before, together with, or in the absence of HTLV-III/LAV-related immunodeficiency.

The animal virus related most closely to HTLV-III/LAV may be a monkey virus discovered in 1985 by M. D. Daniel and his co-workers at the New England Regional Primate Research Center in Southborough, Massachusetts. This virus, simian T-lymphotropic virus type III (STLV-III), was isolated from macaques with immune deficiency syndrome or lymphoma.

The relationship between HTLV-III/LAV and STLV-III is reminiscent of that between HTLV-I and STLV-I (which have more than 95 percent of their nucleotides in common). Some scientists believe that HTLV-III/LAV, like HTLV-I, originated in Africa. They speculate, however, that the AIDS virus jumped species much more recently than the leukemia virus did, perhaps in the 1960s. The African green monkey may have been the source of both viruses. This animal carries STLV-I and STLV-III but, unlike other primates, does not get sick from them. The virus could have entered the human population when monkeys bit hunters who were attempting to capture them for food.

Is there something to be learned from the association of HTLV-III/LAV with the lentivirus family? The lessons may seem discouraging. Frequent mutations of the lentivirus that infects horses—equine infectious anemia virus—allow the virus to evade elimination by the immune system. The disease caused by the visna viruses of sheep has a long and erratic clinical course, which may include progressive paralysis or relapses and remissions. Some infected animals remain healthy but can transmit the disease to other sheep. The caprine arthritis-encephalitis virus of goats does not evoke neutralizing or protective antibodies—antibodies and virus persist in apparent harmony. Efforts to develop vaccines against these animal lentiviruses have been unsuccessful.

The positive side of the association is that past experience with the animal lentiviruses will help AIDS researchers avoid some of the less productive avenues of investigation. Also, lentivirus studies generally have not received high funding priority, in part because they appeared to have little relevance to human disease. The influx of funds occasioned by the AIDS epidemic could accelerate the maturation of existing ideas and help overcome the major stumbling blocks of the past.

Conclusion

Identification of HTLV-III/LAV as the cause of AIDS would not have been possible without the molecular biology, virology, and recombinant DNA technologies developed over the past 20 years. Laboratory analysis of the structure and function of this virus already has produced major dividends, including the development of a rapid screening test to limit the spread of infection through blood products and to identify those at greatest risk of disease.

Researchers in many countries are investigating the life cycle of HTLV-III/LAV to learn exactly how it infects and destroys cells. This information is essential for the development of new therapeutic techniques and for the design of potential vaccines. As scientists learn more about the sequence of events between initial infection and the appearance of AIDS, they may find that certain factors, such as frequent exposure to other viruses or infectious agents (see Chapter 5), increase the likelihood of full-blown disease. Such knowledge could lead to new preventive strategies to help the hundreds of thousands of people already infected with the virus.

Studies of HTLV-III/LAV also will contribute to understanding of how the body functions. Comparisons of the effects of HTLV-I and HTLV-III on T lymphocytes may reveal new facts about the workings of the human immune system and about mechanisms of cell growth and development. And, finally, investigations of how this virus affects nerve cells could increase understanding of other neurological diseases.

* * *

Chapter 4 is based on the presentations of Robert C. Gallo, National Cancer Institute; Richard T. Johnson, Johns Hopkins University School of Medicine; and Luc Montagnier, Institut Pasteur.

5

Damage to the Immune System and the Brain

Confirmation of the role of HTLV-III/LAV in the development of AIDS and AIDS-related conditions opened exciting new avenues of research. Experiments were designed to identify the cells most likely to be affected by the virus and to learn the fate of infected cells in the body. Each new discovery gave scientists a better understanding of the kinds of approaches that would be needed to help AIDS patients and to limit the spread of disease.

After discussing the healthy immune system, the chapter focuses on how HTLV-III/LAV disrupts this system. As noted below, quantitative and qualitative defects in several different cell populations contribute to the AIDS patient's susceptibility to a wide range of infections. The chapter also reviews evidence suggesting that the adoption of improved personal health practices might reduce the risk of developing AIDS and other serious health problems in persons who are infected with HTLV-III/LAV but not yet ill. HTLV-III/LAV activity in the brain is then examined briefly. Scientists are only beginning to understand the extent of this problem, which may have serious implications for the long-term health of high-risk groups and may complicate efforts to develop safe and effective drugs to treat AIDS.

The Healthy Immune System

The human immune system consists of many different kinds of cells actively seeking out and eliminating germs and other foreign substances from the body. In the blood, the majority of defenders are white blood cells called phagocytes. These cells are generalists. They have a primitive recognition system that allows them to bind to, engulf, and destroy a wide range of bacteria, viruses, damaged or infected host cells, and other materials. This process is called phagocytosis. The system is not very efficient, however, and many microorganisms have physical or chemical characteristics that enable them to escape detection or destruction.

Two different adaptive responses have evolved to supplement phagocytosis. Both involve a group of smaller white blood cells called lymphocytes. Lymphocytes originate in the bone marrow and are divided into two distinct classes, B lymphocytes and T lymphocytes. When a B cell is stimulated with an appropriate antigen (a foreign protein or sugar molecule), it divides rapidly into a large population of identical daughter cells. These daughter cells grow into small factories that produce and secrete antibody molecules.

Antibodies act in many different ways: they coat invading bacteria to make them more palatable for digestion by phagocytes, they neutralize bacterial toxins (poisons), and they destroy virus particles or prevent them from binding to target cells. This antibody, or "humoral," immune response is specific. That is, antibodies made against one microorganism will not react against another microorganism unless the two share a common molecular structure.

The second type of adaptive immune response is cell-mediated immunity. The principal actor in this type of reaction is the cytotoxic (cell killing) T lymphocyte. Cell-mediated immunity confers protection against bacteria that live and grow inside host cells (such as the organisms that cause tuberculosis and leprosy) and against certain viruses. Cytotoxic T lymphocytes attack infected cells to prevent the microorganisms inside from replicating and spreading to other sites. Cell-mediated immunity also plays a key role in the rejection of tissue transplants.

Modern techniques in molecular biology have contributed greatly to our knowledge of these adaptive immune responses. For example, scientists have known for many years that animals without T cells cannot mount an effective antibody response against some antigens, even though T cells do not secrete antibodies themselves. In the late 1970s, researchers established that a specific subclass of T cells (identified by a "T4" surface molecule not found on other kinds of T cells) was responsible for this activity. Antibody production depended on cooperation between T4 cells and the appropriate B cells.

Subsequent studies have shown that the T4 cell directly or indirectly regulates every facet of immune function. Anthony S. Fauci, director of the National Institute of Allergy and Infectious Diseases (NIAID), refers to this cell as the "conductor of the symphony of the human immune system." Another way to think of the T4 cell is to imagine it as the dispatcher for a communitywide disaster-response network. This dispatcher takes information about impending emergencies from roving patrol cars and sends out specially trained teams to respond. Without the dispatcher, the flow of information would stop. Individual patrols might be able to handle small problems in the field, but any problem large enough to require a coordinated response would quickly overwhelm the community.

T4 cells coordinate the activities of phagocytes, B lymphocytes, cytotoxic T lymphocytes, and several other immune cells. For example, they produce special chemical messengers that control the movements and function of a group of phagocytic cells in the blood called monocytes. These chemical messengers recruit monocytes to the site of an infection, prevent them from leaving, and stimulate them to kill ingested bacteria or viruses.

As noted above, T4 cells also induce B cells to produce antibodies against some types of antigen. This process actually begins with the monocyte, which predigests the antigen and then presents tiny fragments to an appropriate T4 cell (see Figure 11). The T4 cell, in turn, offers the bits of antigen to a resting B lymphocyte. When the B cell binds to the antigen,

ANTIBODY PRODUCTION

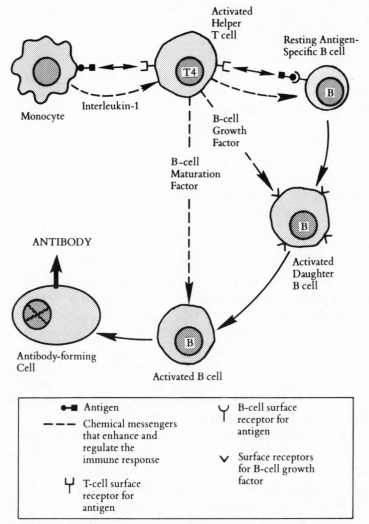

FIGURE 11. Cooperation between T4 cells and antigen-specific B cells in the production of antibody. The helper T cell is activated by interleukin-1 produced during interaction with the antigen-presenting monocyte. The activated T cell then presents the antigen to a resting antigen-specific B cell, which begins to divide. The daughter B cells proliferate extensively under the influence of B-cell growth factor, manufactured by the helper T cell. B-cell maturation factor, also produced by the helper T cell, stops the cell division and turns the activated B cells into antibody-producing cells. Source: Adapted, with permission, from Ivan M. Roitt, *Essential Immunology*, 5th ed. (Oxford: Blackwell Scientific Publications, 1984), Figure 3.16.

the T4 cell produces more chemical messengers that induce the B cell to divide and begin producing antibody.

The T4 cell, again assisted by the monocyte, also regulates cell-mediated immunity against diseases such as herpes and tuberculosis. In this case, T4 cells enhance the activity of cytotoxic T lymphocytes, which carry a T8 surface marker (see Figure 12). The stimulated T8 lymphocytes multiply and attack infected target cells.

Other elements of the immune system regulated by T4 cells include suppressor cells and natural killer cells. Suppressor cells dampen immune reactions to prevent them from damaging healthy tissues. Natural killer cells destroy some types of tumor cells.

Disruption of Immune Function

The first attempts to assess the effects of AIDS on the human immune system resulted in an apparent paradox: the broad range of clinical signs and symptoms associated with the disease suggested multiple problems crippling many facets of the immune response, but a closer look showed a rather selective defect in one component of the system. The explanation, of course, was that the HTLV-III/LAV virus was selectively destroying the T4 lymphocyte (see Figure 13), the dispatcher cell described above.

In most healthy persons, 60 percent of T lymphocytes in the circulation are T4 cells. T8 cells constitute 30 percent, so the T4/T8 ratio is 2. In AIDS patients the number of T4 cells is drastically reduced, so the T4/T8 ratio is much lower than 2 and may even be reversed.

Early in the AIDS epidemic, measurement of the T4/T8 ratio was used by physicians in the diagnosis of AIDS. But other viral infections also can alter this ratio, and some of these infections are common in the populations at risk of AIDS. This created confusion until researchers showed that the effect of HTLV-III/LAV was different from that of the other viruses—the abnormal ratio produced by other viral infections resulted from an increase in T8 cells and not from a decrease in

CELL-MEDIATED IMMUNITY

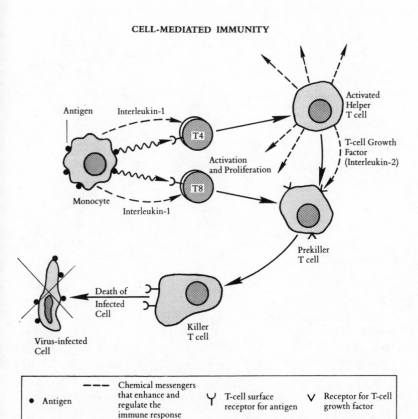

FIGURE 12.   The cell-mediated immune response. Interaction with the antigen-presenting monocyte results in activation of both the T4 cell and the T8 cell. The activated helper T cell produces T-cell growth factor (interleukin-2) and other chemical messengers that lead to proliferation and maturation of the killer T cell (the cytotoxic T lymphocyte). The killer T cell then attacks and destroys the virus-infected target cell. Source: Adapted, with permission, from Ivan M. Roitt, *Essential Immunology*, 5th ed. (Oxford: Blackwell Scientific Publications, 1984), Figures 3.19 and 3.20.

INFECTION WITH HTLV-III/LAV

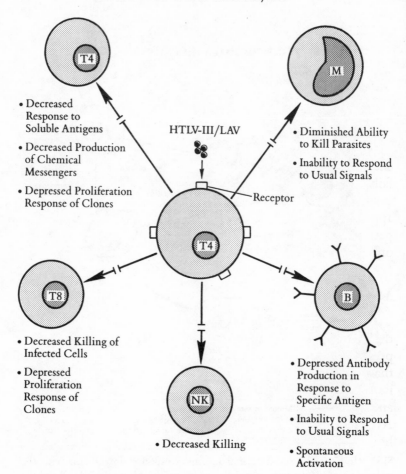

FIGURE 13.   The T4 helper lymphocyte plays a central role in the immune system. This figure shows some of the many functional defects caused by infection of the T4 cell with HTLV-III/LAV. Cells affected include other T cells, B cells, natural killer cells (NK), and monocytes (M). Source: Adapted, with permission, from D. L. Bowen, H. C. Lane, and A. S. Fauci, "Immunopathogenesis of the Acquired Immunodeficiency Syndrome," *Annals of Internal Medicine*, Vol. 103, No. 5 (1985), Figure 3.

T4 cells. The proliferation of T8 cells was determined to be a normal protective mechanism. In contrast, the loss of T4 cells was a sign of serious disease.

T4 cells from AIDS patients also have a major functional defect. They cannot respond to specific antigen. When normal T cells are challenged in a test tube with a protein such as tetanus toxoid, they immediately begin to divide and multiply. Clifford Lane of the NIAID Laboratory of Immunoregulation and his co-workers have shown that T lymphocytes from patients with AIDS do not proliferate after such a challenge. Subsequent experiments demonstrated that this failure to respond is not caused by an inability to divide; it is caused by the inability to recognize antigen. This defect appears early in the disease; it was recognized first in cells from patients with early Kaposi's sarcoma who appeared to have only minor immunologic abnormalities.

Monocyte Defects

Lane and his co-workers recognized the possibility that the failure of T cells to respond might originate in the cells that present antigen to the T lymphocytes (the monocytes), rather than in the T lymphocytes themselves. They explored this issue by challenging different combinations of lymphocytes and monocytes from twin brothers; one twin had full-blown AIDS and the other was healthy. The researchers found that healthy lymphocytes mixed with healthy monocytes responded normally to antigen stimulation, but that none of the other combinations (healthy monocytes and infected lymphocytes, infected monocytes and healthy lymphocytes, or infected monocytes and infected lymphocytes) produced a similar effect.

These experiments indicate that monocytes from AIDS patients also have a specific defect, because they cannot respond normally to the chemical signals of healthy T lymphocytes and they are less able than normal cells are to destroy foreign substances. Preliminary evidence indicates that they, too, may be infected with HTLV-III/LAV. If so, they may be a reservoir of viral infection.

B-Lymphocyte Hyperreactivity

Scientists initially believed that B lymphocytes were not affected by infection with HTLV-III/LAV because patients with AIDS produced normal or higher-than-normal levels of antibodies. New studies have revealed, however, that these high antibody levels do not signify a healthy immune response. Too many B cells are producing antibodies for no apparent reason.

The B-cell population in a healthy person contains cells at three different stages of activation. Some cells are resting and can be induced to divide and multiply by mitogens, substances that stimulate B-cell proliferation without a T-cell intermediary; a second group is partially activated and ready to respond to T-cell signals; and a third group spontaneously secretes antibody.

A 1983 analysis of B-cell populations from 12 patients with AIDS showed that these cells did not follow the pattern described above. Lane and his co-workers reported that the individuals in the study appeared to have no resting B cells; decreased numbers of partially activated cells; and an abnormally high number of fully differentiated, antibody-secreting cells.

The most serious consequence of this hyperreactivity is that the abnormally activated, antibody-secreting B cells in AIDS are not available to respond to signals that trigger a normal humoral response. When a new antigen enters the body, these B cells cannot be recruited to fight it. The disaster-response analogy mentioned earlier is helpful here, too. If all of the specialized response teams were out answering false alarms, they would not be available when an emergency arose that required their unique skills. Similarly, the B cells in AIDS patients are busily producing unnecessary antibodies and are not able to respond when a real need arises.

This hyperreactivity diminishes the ability of AIDS patients to resist disease and also complicates the diagnosis of many opportunistic infections, because the patient does not make detectable antibodies against invading viruses or bacteria. Also, the presence of large quantities of superfluous antibody increases the likelihood of an autoimmune reaction, in which the body begins to attack itself.

The reasons for the abnormal activation of B lymphocytes in AIDS remain unclear. Initially it was thought to result from a co-infection with cytomegalovirus or Epstein-Barr virus; both are present in the majority of AIDS patients, and both have been shown to cause B-cell hyperreactivity. Recent evidence indicates, however, that the AIDS virus itself can trigger such a response.

The Course of Infection in the Body

Early experiments provided information on the characteristics of different cell populations in AIDS patients, but they did not offer a clear picture of how the disease progresses in the body. Thomas Folks of NIAID and his colleagues have developed a laboratory model, using a classic line of T lymphocytes with appropriate T4 markers, that appears to mimic the infection of T4 cells in the natural disease. Their findings have major implications for carriers of HTLV-III/LAV.

The NIAID researchers added HTLV-III/LAV to a previously uninfected culture of T4 cells. The culture grew normally until about the tenth day, when reverse transcriptase activity appeared in the system and cells began to die (as discussed in Chapter 4, reverse transcriptase is the enzyme that transcribes the RNA carried inside each virus particle into the DNA necessary for viral replication). At first it seemed as if the whole culture might succumb, but gradually the reverse transcriptase activity declined and then disappeared. The remaining cells looked and acted healthy, but were they?

Molecular analysis of the surfaces of these cells showed that they were missing the T4 marker. This was an important clue. Folks and his colleagues suspected that the missing markers might indicate a hidden infection, and indeed when they chemically stimulated the cells to divide, reverse transcriptase activity returned and the cells began secreting viruses. In contrast, cells that were not stimulated continued to grow and were not infectious to other cells.

HTLV-III/LAV infection may follow a similar course inside the body. Members of the Sydney AIDS Study Group in Australia described an acute mononucleosis-like syndrome in homosexual men that appeared shortly before the development of antibodies against HTLV-III/LAV. This illness probably corresponds to the initial period of viral replication and loss of lymphocytes seen in the laboratory culture. The Australian researchers suggested that patients might be highly infectious during this acute phase (but only through the routes discussed earlier: intimate sexual practices and needle sharing).

The acute illness lasted up to 14 days in the Australian men and then gradually disappeared (although some of the patients continued to experience mild fevers and other symptoms). Comparison with the cell culture model described above suggests that after recovery from the acute infection, persons who appear healthy may carry a small population of T4 cells that harbor unexpressed or resting HTLV-III/LAV proviruses integrated into their DNA. Months or years later, these proviruses could be turned on to produce large quantities of new virus particles and completely overwhelm any remaining defensive capabilities. The individuals again would become highly infectious and might develop ARC or AIDS.

Fauci and others believe that reinfection with HTLV-III/LAV or infection with another virus might be the trigger that activates the provirus. In the process of switching on transcription mechanisms to fight the new infection, the T cell would turn on the viral genes. This would lead to rapid production of new HTLV-III/LAV particles.

This model may be oversimplified and many aspects of it require additional investigation, but the message for persons who know they are infected with HTLV-III/LAV is clear: avoiding other infections through careful attention to health habits may reduce the risk of developing serious disease. (Theoretically, vaccines also could stimulate infected T cells and lead to the production of new virus particles—infected persons should discuss this possibility with their physicians before receiving any immunizations.)

The Immune System's Response

How does the immune system fight back when it is attacked by HTLV-III/LAV? Most patients with AIDS or ARC and many persons at high risk for the syndrome make detectable levels of antibodies against some of the HTLV-III/LAV viral proteins. The problem is that most of these antibodies are not capable of neutralizing or destroying the virus. Few studies have been undertaken to determine if there is a correlation between a patient's clinical status and the type or quantity of antibodies produced.

Robert C. Gallo and his co-workers at the National Cancer Institute report that they can now isolate active virus from the blood of more than 80 percent of those who have antibodies against HTLV-III/LAV. Researchers at New England Deaconess Hospital in Boston, in collaboration with the NCI scientists, have found that a small proportion of apparently healthy homosexuals and heterosexual partners of AIDS patients test negative for antibody and positive for virus. One of the major research challenges for the future will be to sort out these complexities and to develop a better understanding of the antibody response to this infection.

Preliminary studies by Fauci and his co-workers indicate that both antibodies and cytotoxic T cells from patients infected with HTLV-III/LAV are capable of destroying virus-infected T4 cells in the laboratory. While the clinical implications of this work remain unclear, efforts are under way to determine how the information provided by these studies can be exploited in the development of preventive and therapeutic techniques (see Chapter 6).

Infection in the Brain

Following the discovery of HTLV-III/LAV, researchers at the National Cancer Institute and other laboratories de-

signed chemical probes to hunt for the virus in cells throughout the body. One of their first findings was that cells in the
brains of some AIDS patients showed unmistakable signs of
productive virus infection. In fact, the number of infected cells
in the brain appeared higher than that in the blood.

Diseases of the central nervous system had been recognized as an important facet of the AIDS problem since the
beginning of the epidemic. Well-defined lesions, such as those
caused by tumors and certain parasitic diseases (see Chapter 3),
were identified in some patients. Many others, however,
showed signs of a more widespread degeneration of the brain
that could not be traced to any specific cause. These patients
initially experienced mild memory loss or problems controlling body movements, but the symptoms often progressed to
severe dementia or paralysis.

The physicians treating these patients first thought that
they were simply missing or misinterpreting the signs of a
familiar organism, but as the number of cases mounted they
became suspicious. If the immune defects associated with
AIDS were caused by an infectious agent, perhaps the same
agent was affecting the brain. The discovery of HTLV-
III/LAV in cells within the brain confirmed this hypothesis.

Some researchers believe that the brain cells infected with
HTLV-III/LAV are glial cells. These cells provide structural
support to nerve cells, help regulate the transfer of nutrients
from blood vessels to nerve tissues, and act like blood
phagocytes by removing cellular debris from the brain.

The discovery of HTLV-III/LAV within the brain has
caused growing concern for several reasons. First, it suggests
a closer relationship to retroviruses that cause neurological
disease in other animals, such as the visna virus in sheep. A
related issue involves the length of the incubation period, the
time between infection and onset of symptomatic disease. The
Centers for Disease Control has estimated a mean incubation
period of $4\frac{1}{2}$ years for transfusion-associated AIDS. But the
mean incubation period for some other slow virus diseases of
the brain approaches 15 years. The true incubation period for
HTLV-III/LAV infection may not be known for several
decades.

The discovery of the virus in the brain also has important therapeutic implications. Various techniques have been proposed to remove virus from the blood and restore the immune system, but if brain cells continue producing virus, any improvements attained with these techniques probably would be temporary. Successful therapy will require a drug that can pass through the physiologic barrier between the bloodstream and the brain and that is nontoxic to brain tissues.

Finally, the association between AIDS and neurological impairment may increase the impact of the disease on the health care system in the United States. The potential needs of a large patient population with both major physical problems and severe cognitive disabilities could prove overwhelming for some medical facilities.

Conclusion

HTLV-III/LAV infection produces a broad spectrum of immunologic abnormalities, but the principal cause of these abnormalities appears to be the progressive destruction of one subclass of T lymphocytes. These helper cells, identified by a T4 surface molecule, play a central role in all the body's major defense mechanisms. Patients who have relatively low T4 levels appear to be more susceptible to opportunistic infections than those with higher levels.

In addition to this quantitative defect, researchers have identified a variety of functional defects both in T4 lymphocytes and in other components of the immune system in AIDS. A T4 cell infected with HTLV-III/LAV appears to lose its ability to respond to specific antigens. In addition, the virus serves as a B-cell activator: B cells from AIDS patients spontaneously proliferate and secrete antibodies, thus becoming unable to respond to the signals that evoke a normal antibody response. Monocytes from these patients also are defective; they exhibit a diminished ability to respond to chemical signals and to destroy certain parasites.

Laboratory models of AIDS infection suggest that health status may play an important role in both susceptibility to infection and the development of serious disease. Scientists

believe that a subsequent infection's activation of a lymphocyte harboring an HTLV-III/LAV provirus may trigger the
production of new viruses and lead to the development of
clinical symptoms.

The body's response to HTLV-III/LAV remains poorly
understood. Almost all infected persons make antibodies
against the virus, but these antibodies generally are not protective. Further, researchers have isolated active virus from
some apparently healthy individuals without antibodies. More
studies need to be undertaken to determine the relationship
between the type and quantity of antibodies produced and the
patient's clinical status.

The discovery of HTLV-III/LAV in the brain has several
potentially serious implications for healthy individuals infected with the virus, for AIDS patients, and for the health
care system as a whole. Similarities between the AIDS virus
and retroviruses that infect the brain in other animals suggest
that the incubation period may be longer than previously
suspected and that more of those infected eventually may
succumb to the disease. The discovery of HTLV-III/LAV in
the brain also helps explain the severe neurological problems
and depression seen in some AIDS patients.

*   *   *

Chapter 5 is based on the presentations of Anthony S. Fauci,
National Institute of Allergy and Infectious Diseases; Robert C.
Gallo, National Cancer Institute; Richard T. Johnson, Johns Hop-
kins University School of Medicine; and Luc Montagnier, Institut
Pasteur.

6

Prevention and Treatment

In an era when many young physicians have never seen a case of measles or polio and when once life-threatening bacterial infections disappear in two or three days with antibiotic therapy, the AIDS epidemic seems almost unreal. The temptation to believe that a vaccine or a miracle drug is just over the horizon may be overwhelming for both health care providers and the general public. But public health experts warn that the United States cannot wait for a medical solution to the AIDS crisis—the rapid increase in cases necessitates immediate action.

More than 90 percent of AIDS cases have been attributed to high-risk sexual behavior or intravenous drug abuse. Control of the epidemic depends on education and other public health measures to change these behaviors. Preventive measures must be carefully tailored to address the needs of high-risk groups as well as the concerns of the general populace. As the infection spreads, it is crucial that messages about risk reduction reach as wide an audience as possible.

This emphasis on prevention is not meant to detract from the efforts of hundreds of scientists in the United States and abroad who are exploring new therapeutic approaches to HTLV-III/LAV infection, described in the last half of the chapter. Never has the scientific community responded so quickly to a new medical problem. The development of safe and effective drugs takes time, however; researchers have just begun to understand how to fight chronic viral infections of

89

any kind. Scientists searching for an AIDS vaccine also face many obstacles, and even if they develop a suitable candidate, the logistics of clinical trials and the complexities of liability issues may delay adoption of such a vaccine for a decade or longer. Until antiviral therapy and a vaccine are ready for widespread use, education and other public health measures are the only weapons against AIDS.

Education and Other Public Health Measures

Risk-reduction education to control AIDS must be based on the assumption that public health education works, even in areas as sensitive as lifelong sexual behavior, although evidence about the validity of this assumption is mixed. Americans generally do not have a very good record with respect to diseases that require long-term behavioral changes. People of all ages continue to smoke despite the clear connection between smoking and lung cancer. Alcohol problems and dietary habits linked to heart disease are equally resistant to change.

The desire to avoid HTLV-III/LAV infection may be stronger, however, because the problem is new and because its most familiar manifestation, AIDS, is uniformly fatal. The dramatic decrease in the incidence of rectal gonorrhea and other sexually transmitted diseases among homosexual men in this country is one indication that members of this high-risk population have responded to local educational campaigns. (The data on gonorrhea do not give a clear picture of the extent or nature of these behavioral changes, however, because the relationship between sexual activity and disease transmission is complicated by many other factors.)

To learn more about how different sectors of the homosexual community have responded to the AIDS crisis, several research groups have conducted telephone and written surveys focusing on changes in sexual behavior. Overall, they have found that homosexual men tend to have fewer sexual partners and are less likely to engage in high-risk activities (such as sex with strangers, anal intercourse without a condom, and oral sex with exchange of semen) than they were in the past.

These behavior changes have not been uniform, however. Leon McKusick of the University of California at San Francisco and his colleagues have developed a partial profile of those who are least likely to reduce their number of sexual contacts. They are older men whose first homosexual experience was many years ago, men not involved in monogamous relationships, and men who do not have a visual image of someone in the advanced stages of AIDS deterioration. Information such as that provided by the profile will contribute to the development of better educational campaigns for high-risk groups.

Gauging the potential success of AIDS education programs for the general public is more difficult, in part because of the social taboo against talking openly about sexually transmitted diseases. Very little information is available about the effectiveness of health education in limiting the spread of these diseases within the heterosexual population.

The urgency of the AIDS problem further complicates the development of appropriate public information efforts. Researchers structuring antismoking or weight reduction campaigns have time to try out their materials on small groups, analyze the results, and make needed revisions. When the problems addressed are reversible, such delays probably do not have a major impact on public health. But infection with HTLV-III/LAV is not reversible. The challenge for government and community organizations is to develop innovative approaches to AIDS education that are flexible enough to change as new information becomes available.

Reaching High-Risk Groups

This section focuses on broad efforts to change behavior within specific risk groups. Voluntary testing and counseling for individuals are discussed in the following section.

Homosexuals   Some of the most effective public information campaigns on AIDS have been carried out in San Francisco, a city with a large homosexual population. Several factors have contributed to the success of these educational programs, according to Mervyn F. Silverman, the city's former Director of Health. The first has been cooperation. From the beginning of the epidemic, public health officials have worked closely with organizations representing high-risk groups and with the local medical community. This sharing of information has prevented the dissemination of conflicting messages that could have caused serious confusion.

The second factor in this success was early realization by the organizations involved that educational campaigns for high-risk groups have to be specific. Simply stating that sexual intercourse increases the risk of AIDS is not enough, because it is unlikely that those worried about AIDS will stop having sex altogether. The messages have to be explicit about which activities to avoid and how to have sexual contact without transferring the virus.

A good example of this concept is the brochure called *AIDS and Healthful Gay Sexual Activity* produced by the American Association of Physicians for Human Rights (AAPHR), the national association of homosexual physicians. One section of the brochure focuses on decreasing the number of sexual partners, the use of condoms, and avoidance of substance abuse. Another section, entitled "Positive Steps You Should Take," urges readers to ask about the health of sex partners; to increase touching and caressing; to check partners for swollen glands or skin sores and spots; and to get adequate rest, nutrition, and exercise. The recommendation for those who know or suspect that they have AIDS or ARC is "don't risk the health of others by having sex. Be sensible. Consult a health care provider who is up to date on gay health care."

Materials similar to the AAPHR brochure are available through AIDS hotlines or action centers in most major cities in the United States.

The provision of educational materials on AIDS by state and local health departments varies, in part because some policymakers and segments of the lay public believe that it is unacceptable for a government agency to provide advice about "safe sex" for homosexuals. (This issue is discussed further in Chapter 8.)

Another lesson from the San Francisco experience is that efforts to promote changes in behavior (such as reducing the number of sexual partners) are most effective at limiting the spread of disease in areas where the prevalence of infection is low. If a large proportion of a community has been infected, substantial reductions in high-risk behaviors may not be enough to slow the epidemic. This fact, combined with the long latency period characteristic of AIDS, suggests that communities should not delay public information programs for high-risk populations until the problem in their area gets worse. The time to begin these programs is before the virus becomes widespread in a community.

Intravenous Drug Abusers   As stated earlier, AIDS poses a major threat to the health of intravenous drugs abusers, their sexual partners, and their children. More than two-thirds of AIDS cases resulting from heterosexual intercourse with a member of a recognized high-risk group involve sexual contact with an intravenous drug abuser. More than half of all children with AIDS have at least one parent who is a drug abuser.

Transmission of HTLV-III/LAV among drug abusers results from sharing hypodermic needles and syringes. Options proposed to reduce this practice include (1) decreasing the amount of illegal drug abuse generally, (2) providing sterile needles and syringes (through public or private agencies), and (3) educating drug users about sterilization procedures and the need to seek out and pay for clean equipment.

The first option is a laudable long-term goal, but neither stricter law enforcement nor increased availability of legal alternatives, such as methadone maintenance, is likely to produce the immediate reduction in numbers of injections required to slow the spread of HTLV-III/LAV.

The second option, the provision of sterile equipment, has been adopted quietly by some European countries, but in the United States the concept has aroused considerable controversy. Most arguments focus on the moral dilemma raised when government organizations provide the materials necessary to carry out an illegal act. Those in favor of the distribution of clean needles and syringes counter that the public health risk presented by AIDS justifies changing the rules.

Many public health officials believe that the final option, risk-reduction education for intravenous drug abusers, is unrealistic because the target population simply will not listen. Yet, Don C. Des Jarlais and his co-workers from the New York State Division of Substance Abuse Services and Narcotic and Drug Research, Inc., report "universal awareness of AIDS among intravenous drug users in New York and a sustained reduction in needle sharing." Concern over the disease also has produced increased demand for new, unused needles. (This, in turn, has led to the detrimental practice of selling "resealed" needles—sellers on the street put used, unsterilized needles back into their original wrappings, reseal them, and sell them again.) These findings indicate that risk reduction already has begun among intravenous drug abusers in response to the AIDS epidemic.

Des Jarlais and his colleagues suggest that as members of this population come to understand the full impact of infection with HTLV-III/LAV (especially that it can increase susceptibility even to diseases that are not now covered by the CDC definition of AIDS, such as tuberculosis), they might become more receptive to public health efforts.

Public health messages targeted for intravenous drug abusers and the communities in which they live should contain two recommendations in addition to a warning against sharing needles. The first is that condoms should be used to prevent transmission of the virus from infected to uninfected sexual partners. The second is that women who use intravenous drugs or whose sexual partners are drug abusers should postpone pregnancy until more is known about AIDS.

Hemophiliacs   AIDS in the third major high-risk group in the United States, hemophiliacs, is not a consequence of life-style choices—it is not a behavioral disease. Nevertheless, hemophiliacs must take the same precautions to prevent transmission of HTLV-III/LAV as others who have been exposed to the virus. The National Hemophilia Foundation produces a variety of educational materials about AIDS for hemophiliacs, their families, and health care providers. (These materials are available through local chapters of the foundation or from the national office in New York City.) Hemophiliacs and their sexual partners are urged to adopt practices that minimize the exchange of body fluids during sexual intercourse and to consider delaying having children until more is known about the syndrome.

Voluntary Testing and Counseling for Individuals at High Risk

Information is the most important resource for members of high-risk groups concerned about the risk of AIDS (see Appendix E for a list of national organizations offering information on AIDS). These persons should take advantage of local and national AIDS hotlines and confidential community counseling services to learn as much as possible about the factors that increase and decrease risk.

In March 1986 the Public Health Service (PHS) recommended that persons at increased risk of HTLV-III/LAV infection undergo periodic blood tests to determine whether they have become infected with the virus. To ensure the availability of these tests, the PHS also recommended that counseling and voluntary blood testing be offered routinely to these individuals when they seek medical care (see Appendix C). PHS officials stress that efforts to increase the number of persons requesting such testing and counseling will depend on the ability of health departments to assure confidentiality and to protect records from any unauthorized disclosure.

The recommendations specify that persons at increased risk include (1) homosexual and bisexual men; (2) present or past intravenous drug users; (3) persons with clinical or laboratory evidence of infection, such as those with signs or symptoms compatible with AIDS or ARC; (4) persons born in countries where heterosexual transmission is thought to play a major role (for example, Haiti and central African countries); (5) male or female prostitutes and their sex partners; (6) sex partners of infected persons or persons at increased risk; (7) all persons with hemophilia who have received clotting-factor products; (8) newborn infants of high-risk or infected mothers.

Many individuals who consider themselves at risk of AIDS already have been tested at one of the special antibody testing sites funded originally through the CDC. These alternative antibody testing sites were established in response to concerns that once blood banks began screening donated blood for HTLV-III/LAV antibodies, some members of high-risk groups (who previously had followed recommendations to refrain from blood donation) might be tempted to donate blood solely to learn their antibody status. Because the screening test is not 100 percent accurate, this might have had the paradoxical effect of increasing transfusion-associated AIDS. At a time when few laboratories outside blood banks were equipped to screen for HTLV-III/LAV antibodies, the alternative testing sites permitted high-risk individuals to find out their antibody status without entering the blood-donor pool. (Today, the antibody screening test is available at many public health facilities.)

Most public health officials support voluntary use of the HTLV-III/LAV antibody test by high-risk individuals. They believe that a positive test result encourages an individual to adopt behavioral practices that reduce the risk of future health problems and that limit the spread of infection to others. (Appendix C contains recommendations for counseling high-risk persons who test both positive and negative.)

Until recently, the AAPHR discouraged homosexual men from obtaining the test. The association's position was based on two factors: (1) concern that despite procedures to maintain confidentiality, test results could become available to employers, insurance companies, or others who might use them as a basis for discrimination; and (2) the conviction that science has nothing to offer those who test positive. The current AAPHR position is that taking the test is an individual decision—those who feel they need to know their antibody status to effect a change in behavior should take the test—but only where it is offered anonymously and with appropriate pre- and post-test counseling. As explained by an AAPHR spokesman, a fundamental element of the association's views on antibody testing is that, regardless of test results, all homosexual men should behave as if they and their sexual partners carry the virus. In other words, they should follow guidelines for safe and sensible sex and refrain from donating blood, semen, or organs for transplantation.

AIDS Cofactors   Although it is true that scientists still know very little about why some people infected with HTLV-III/LAV develop AIDS and why other infected individuals have milder symptoms or remain healthy, laboratory studies have provided some clues about susceptibility (see Chapter 5). The most important is that an immune system besieged by multiple infections may be more likely to succumb to the effects of HTLV-III/LAV.

This means that individuals who have been exposed to the virus or who are concerned about exposure should take steps to maintain good general health: they should eat regularly, exercise, get enough sleep, and reduce stress levels through counseling or other means. They also should avoid activities that interfere with good judgment, such as abuse of alcohol and drugs (including noninjectable drugs). These recommendations may not prevent AIDS, but they will increase the body's ability to fight infection.

Persons who know they are infected with HTLV-III/LAV also should consult their physicians before receiving any immunizations. Theoretically, stimulation of infected immune cells by a vaccine could lead to the production of new virus particles. Also, an immune system weakened by HTLV-III/LAV might be overwhelmed by the weakened or attenuated live viruses present in some common vaccines.

Recently, nitrite inhalants or "poppers" (used predominantly by homosexuals to enhance sexual experiences) have been suggested as having a role in the development of Kaposi's sarcoma among homosexuals infected with HTLV-III/LAV. Further research is needed to validate these findings.

Government Initiatives: Beyond Voluntary Measures

The March 1986 PHS recommendations focus primarily on education and voluntary testing, but they also express support for state and local actions to regulate or close establishments "where there is evidence that they facilitate high-risk behaviors, such as anonymous sexual contacts and/or intercourse with multiple partners or IV drug abuse (e.g., bathhouses, houses of prostitution, 'shooting galleries')."

This statement of support reflects the fact that potential public health measures cover a wide spectrum of activities—from general education to regulations concerning mandatory testing and quarantine. As measures become more restrictive, public health officials face increasingly complex decisions regarding the balance between a state's right to protect the health of its citizens and the fundamental civil rights of an infected individual. This potential conflict is discussed further in Chapter 8.

Concern that education campaigns may not be sufficient to reduce the spread of AIDS has led public health officials in some states to propose the use of case-finding and contact-tracing methods to control the epidemic. These methods involve interviewing patients with AIDS (or with a positive HTLV-III/LAV antibody test) to obtain the names of sexual contacts, and then testing the contacts to determine whether or not they have been infected. This approach has been used for decades to contain the spread of syphilis.

Colorado became the first state to take steps toward contact tracing in the fall of 1985, when its Board of Health voted to require laboratories to report each confirmed positive test for HTLV-III/LAV antibodies with the name and address of the patient and the attending physician. State officials say that the main purpose of the program is individual education—to ensure that all those with positive test results receive skilled follow-up and counseling, either from their own physicians or from health department staff, about the risk of transmitting the disease to others. They anticipate that contact tracing will be used in a relatively small proportion of cases, for example, in situations involving bisexual males who may transmit the virus to wives of childbearing age. They emphasize that all patient information will be handled with strict confidentiality.

Opponents of such a program argue that contact tracing is not advisable with HTLV-III/LAV infection for several reasons. They are concerned that the potential for abuse of confidentiality rules is too great, especially given the discrimination experienced by many AIDS and ARC patients. In addition, they believe that contact tracing would discourage voluntary use of the blood test.

Risk-Reduction Education for the General Population

The incidence of HTLV-III/LAV infection in the general population has remained extremely low. This is encouraging, but it also means that the low-risk heterosexual population may be less responsive to risk-reduction advice than members of high-risk groups. Unquestionably, a person who has watched several friends battle a fatal disease is more likely to take advice about avoiding the disease than someone who has no personal experience with it.

Another factor that complicates information and education efforts for the general population is that different audiences require very different types of materials. A parent who is worried about the presence of a child with AIDS in the local elementary school, for example, has concerns different from those of the sexually active high school or college student.

The U.S. Public Health Service has produced guidelines advising communities how to deal with AIDS in the classroom (Appendix D) and in the workplace (Appendix B). Both sets of guidelines stress that AIDS is not spread by the types of nonsexual, person-to-person contacts likely to occur in schools, offices, and factories. In general, elementary school children and adolescents with AIDS whose physicians believe they are well enough to attend school should be permitted to do so without restrictions. The PHS guidelines recommend that decisions about school attendance be made by using the team approach—including the child's physician and parent or guardian, public health personnel, and personnel associated with the proposed care or educational setting.

Infected preschool-aged children and older children with AIDS who for some reason are unable to control their body secretions, are prone to biting, or have open sores may pose a risk to others. These children should be placed in more restricted school or day care settings. The PHS recommendations provide special guidelines for persons caring for these children (Appendix D). All schools and day care facilities should adopt routine procedures for handling blood and other body fluids whether or not children with HTLV-III/LAV are enrolled.

There is no evidence of transmission of AIDS in personal-service settings such as barbershops and beauty salons. Workers in these fields are advised, however, that transmission theoretically could occur in the highly unlikely event that copious amounts of blood from a person infected with HTLV-III/LAV came into contact with an open wound in another person.

Services such as ear piercing and tattooing that involve intentional breakage of the skin may involve a small risk of infection if needles and other tools are not sterilized properly. Clients should assess the cleanliness of the establishment in which these services are provided and should ask about sterilization practices before undergoing the procedures.

Precautions for health care workers (Appendix B) focus on the proper handling and disposal of needles, syringes, and other sharp objects. (The few documented work-related infections with HTLV-III/LAV in health care settings have involved needle sticks or other puncture wounds with equipment previously used on an AIDS patient.) Hospital and emergency personnel also should use special care in administering mouth-to-mouth cardiopulmonary resuscitation (CPR) to AIDS patients and to others who may be infected with HTLV-III/LAV, although there is no evidence that the disease has been transmitted in this way. Resuscitation bags or disposable devices to prevent mouth-to-mouth contact between the resuscitator and the patient should be used if available.

Fear of AIDS has led some members of the general public to postpone health care procedures such as dental surgery and eye examinations. Although there is no evidence to date that the virus has been transmitted through medical instruments, the Centers for Disease Control has issued guidelines to ensure that all personnel in these areas understand and follow proper sterilization techniques. These techniques completely eliminate the risk of transmission of HTLV-III/LAV from one patient to another.

Concern about AIDS also has led some surgical patients to insist upon choosing their own blood donors from among family and friends. Such designated donation is firmly opposed by the American Red Cross and by the other major voluntary blood-donor organizations. Several studies have shown that the incidence of HTLV-III/LAV infection among designated donors is no lower than that among volunteer blood donors; in fact, family pressure to donate blood for a sick relative may lead some persons to ignore their high-risk status and donate blood when they would not do so otherwise. Donor screening and routine testing of all donated blood and blood products for HTLV-III/LAV antibodies have reduced the risk of transfusion-associated AIDS to infinitesimal levels. The use of designated donors does not reduce the risk any further.

Another common misconception, which arose after the discovery of transfusion-associated AIDS, was that people could contract AIDS by donating blood. It is impossible to get AIDS by giving blood because in this country a new, sterilized needle is used for each donor and is then discarded. Misconceptions about blood donation have created intermittent blood shortages across the nation.

Because many teenagers experiment with sex and intravenous drugs, education programs designed to help them make informed decisions about these behaviors are especially important. Existing programs have had mixed results, but the increasing prevalence of AIDS makes such programs more desirable than ever before.

Secondary schools in New York City and other areas where the incidence of AIDS is high have begun to integrate

AIDS education into their curriculums, but much more needs to be done. Colleges and universities also must help their students understand the consequences of infection with HTLV-III/LAV and provide accurate guidelines on risk reduction for the individual.

The principal messages will be the same as those delivered in existing programs: intravenous drug abuse carries a variety of serious health risks, sexual intercourse should be reserved for caring relationships between two people who know each other well, and steps should be taken to prevent the spread of venereal disease. But the threat of AIDS and related diseases necessitates a more direct approach—clear guidelines could save the lives of those who decide to experiment despite the risk. Such guidelines should include the following:

• Shared needles and syringes can transmit AIDS.
• All intravenous drug abusers should be presumed to be potentially infective.
• Because most of those infected with HTLV-III/LAV do not have symptoms, physical appearance should not be used to assess infectivity.
• Prostitutes may become infected with HTLV-III/LAV through intravenous drug abuse or through sexual contact with a member of a high-risk group. Prostitutes should be avoided.
• Picking up strangers and having multiple sex partners increase the risk of infection for heterosexuals as well as homosexuals.
• Anyone engaging in sexual activity except in a long-term, monogamous relationship should use condoms to minimize the exchange of bodily fluids. (Although condoms have not been proved effective at limiting the transmission of AIDS, they have been shown to prevent the passage of HTLV-III/LAV in the laboratory and they do reduce the spread of other sexually transmitted diseases.)
• Although HTLV-III/LAV has been found in the saliva of some patients with AIDS-related complex, there are no documented cases in which kissing has been responsible for transmission of the virus. Nonetheless, deep kissing should be

reserved for long-term relationships in which partners know each other well. Dry or social kissing presents no danger of infection.

School districts and local public health departments will have to match the information presented to the needs and maturity of the audiences involved. Designing programs that provide useful information without causing unwarranted alarm may be difficult, but no community can afford to wait.

Treatment

No one knows how many of the million or more Americans infected with HTLV-III/LAV will eventually become ill, but the need for an effective antiviral treatment becomes more urgent each year. AIDS patients with opportunistic infections and cancers respond poorly to established therapies and have frequent relapses because the virus incapacitates the body's defense mechanisms. HTLV-III/LAV infection and destruction of brain cells may present an even greater threat to the long-term well-being of affected populations.

The search for drugs to control or reduce the impact of the virus has generated cautious optimism among researchers. Several different types of agents inhibit HTLV-III/LAV in the test tube, but the road from laboratory studies to clinical practice is often long and arduous. Only through carefully monitored clinical trials can scientists determine which drugs are both effective and safe enough for long-term use.

In some respects, the outlook for an AIDS therapy is much brighter than it would have been just a decade ago. Historically, medical science has not fared well in the battle against chronic viral infections such as herpes and hepatitis B. But new techniques in virology, cell culture, and molecular biology have begun to turn the tide. Treatments for herpes, papilloma virus (the wart virus), and cytomegalovirus infections have shown promise in extensive clinical trials. In a few cases antiviral agents appear to produce a cure; in most, however, they shorten or prevent the acute signs of infection without eliminating the virus from the body.

Several characteristics of HTLV-III/LAV make it a particularly difficult target. The major complication is that the virus inserts itself into the genetic machinery of infected cells. Before the discovery that the virus replicates in nerve tissues, some researchers believed that it might be possible to eradicate the disease by destroying all infected cells in the body (only a small proportion of immune cells are carrying the virus at any one time). But this strategy may not be feasible for a virus that infects the brain. The most practical goal appears to be to suppress viral replication and prevent the infection of new cells.

Thus, any drugs designed to control AIDS must cross the blood–brain barrier and must be safe enough for lifetime therapy. Moreover, these medications should be suitable for oral use. The need for regular intravenous administration or even intramuscular injections would tie millions of people permanently to the nation's medical institutions. Such restrictions would have an adverse effect on the quality of life for the individual besides overwhelming the health care system. The need for a low-cost, oral drug is even more urgent in developing countries.

Another characteristic of HTLV-III/LAV that complicates therapy is its penchant for the T4 lymphocyte, the master regulator of the human immune system. Researchers involved in developing and testing therapies for other chronic viral infections have found that the immune status of the patient is a crucial factor in the success or failure of treatment. In AIDS the immune system is severely depleted; thus, it is not surprising that transplant patients, in whom physicians can regulate the level of immunosuppression, respond much better to therapy for cytomegalovirus pneumonia and other severe viral infections than do AIDS patients.

Preliminary trials of potential antiviral agents indicate that suppression of the virus alone may not be enough to protect AIDS patients from opportunistic infections and other problems. Although the virus infects only a small number of cells at any one time, it appears to set in motion processes that prevent other immune cells from functioning normally. This effect may remain even after the virus is suppressed.

Another factor hampering clinical research efforts is the

lack of an easily detectable marker to measure HTLV–III/LAV levels in the body. Without such a marker it is very difficult to determine whether an experimental drug is having an effect on the magnitude of a positive response. Markers for hepatitis B virus in the blood and cytomegalovirus in the urine tell researchers within 24 hours whether a patient is responding to a particular course of treatment. In contrast, measurements of HTLV-III/LAV levels take days or even weeks because they depend upon the isolation and growth of the virus in tissue culture systems, an extremely difficult and time-consuming procedure. (Measurement of antibody levels is not suitable for the purpose of monitoring therapy.)

The severity of AIDS and the rapid spread of infection have generated increasing pressure to use antiviral agents before they have been fully tested. Researchers argue that widespread acquiescence to these demands would be short-sighted—only through well-designed clinical trials can scientists determine which agents actually work. This is especially true when the opponent is a viral infection that causes a wide range of clinical symptoms, some of which come and go spontaneously.

The development of a new therapeutic drug begins with laboratory studies to show that it has the potential to suppress or inactivate the infective agent without causing excessive damage to healthy tissues. These studies are conducted in cell cultures and in suitable animal models. If laboratory results are favorable, the investigator requests permission from the Food and Drug Administration (FDA) to begin the first of three phases of clinical trials. Phase I usually involves only a small number of volunteers; the goals are to establish the drug's safety in humans and to begin determination of appropriate dose levels and routes of administration. In phase II trials researchers gather additional information about the most effective way to administer the drug and about possible adverse effects, and they begin to assess its clinical potential. Phase III clinical trials are controlled field studies with larger numbers of patients to develop reasonable estimates of safety and efficacy.

Two approaches have been used by scientists in the

United States and abroad to accelerate the development of anti-AIDS drugs without bypassing established testing procedures. The first has been to examine the susceptibility of HTLV-III/LAV to drugs originally developed for other purposes. The benefit of this approach is that researchers can bypass toxicity studies in animal models and some of the early stages of clinical trials because they already know how the drug affects human tissues.

The second approach has been to develop rapid screening systems for new chemical agents, followed by carefully monitored laboratory and early clinical studies of any promising candidates. In the United States this process has been characterized by ongoing collaborations involving scientists from the National Cancer Institute, the National Institute of Allergy and Infectious Diseases, numerous academic medical centers, and the pharmaceutical industry. Constant communication between research scientists and the FDA has accelerated this process even further.

Drugs Developed for Other Purposes

A variety of existing antiviral drugs have been found to inhibit HTLV-III/LAV in the laboratory, but clinical results have been discouraging. Although some have been shown to reduce viral replication in patients with AIDS, they do not seem to alter the course of disease—the patients keep getting sicker. That may be because most patients enrolled in these early clinical trials were severely ill at the time of treatment—their immune systems may have been beyond repair by available techniques. To be effective, antiviral therapy for HTLV-III/LAV may need to start very early in the course of infection.

This requirement adds another constraint to the search for appropriate drugs. Physicians usually are hesitant to administer drugs to persons who are clinically well, but they may have no choice in this case. Also, healthy individuals are unlikely to comply with a drug regimen that has even minor side effects. Thus, acceptable agents will have to be relatively or absolutely nontoxic.

Suramin   The drug suramin has been used widely in Africa to treat parasitic diseases (trypanosomiasis and onchocerciasis). Its ability to inhibit animal retroviruses was first reported in 1979 by Erik De Clercq of the University of Leuven, Belgium. Suramin, like the majority of antiviral agents employed against HTLV-III/LAV, acts by inhibiting reverse transcriptase, the enzyme that triggers the first step in the virus's natural cycle of replication (see Chapter 4). Figure 14, a schematic diagram of a cell infected with HTLV-III/LAV, shows the possible sites of action of reverse transcriptase inhibitors and other antiviral drugs.

The first reported clinical trial of suramin in patients infected with HTLV-III/LAV involved 6 patients with Kaposi's sarcoma and 4 with ARC. All 10 patients received seven doses over five weeks. By the end of therapy, viral activity had decreased markedly in the 4 patients who had had evidence of HTLV-III/LAV replication before treatment (in 3 cases viral activity was undetectable); but in all cases it returned after the suramin was stopped. No significant clinical or immunologic improvement was observed in any of the patients. Side effects associated with the five-week therapy included fevers, rashes, urinary abnormalities, and transient changes in liver enzymes. The researchers concluded that the results provided a rationale for cautious, experimental trials over longer periods.

Further testing of suramin has revealed a high incidence of adrenal insufficiency among patients treated with the drug. In addition, some studies have suggested that in certain patients the drug might result in an acceleration of the disease. Another drawback of suramin therapy for HTLV-III/LAV infection is the drug's inability to cross the blood–brain barrier.

Interferons   Interferons are natural substances that inhibit a wide spectrum of RNA and DNA viruses. Alpha interferon has been shown to be effective against various types of herpes infections, hepatitis B, and laryngeal warts. In addition, several research teams report that alpha interferon produced by recombinant DNA technology causes regression of Kaposi's sarcoma lesions in some AIDS patients. Controlled

PREVENTING REPLICATION OF HTLV-III/LAV

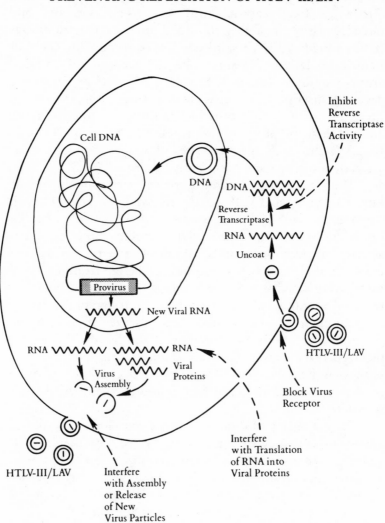

FIGURE 14.   Several of the antiviral drugs now being evaluated for use against HTLV-III/LAV act by inhibiting reverse transcriptase activity. Other possible strategies for preventing replication of the virus include blocking specific cellular receptors for the virus, interfering with translation of viral RNA into new viral proteins, and interfering with the assembly or release of new virus particles.

clinical trials are under way to compare the effects of high-dose interferon, low-dose interferon, and a placebo (an inert substance) in AIDS and ARC patients.

Researchers believe that interferon acts against HTLV-III/LAV by interrupting the formation and release of new virus particles (see Figure 14). Adverse reactions to interferon therapy include fever, reversible bone marrow suppression, and, less commonly, effects on the brain, the liver, and possibly the heart.

Foscarnet First synthesized in 1924, foscarnet (trisodium phosphonoformate) has been evaluated primarily by European researchers as a treatment for herpes infections. Like suramin, it inhibits reverse transcriptase activity. Foscarnet has been shown to block replication of HTLV-III/LAV in the laboratory; clinical trials are under way.

Clinical doses of foscarnet appear to be nontoxic. The drawback of this drug is that it must be given intravenously, which makes it unsuitable for long-term maintenance.

Ribavirin The drug ribavirin inhibits a wide variety of RNA and DNA viruses. Different forms of the drug have been evaluated in the treatment of Lassa fever in West Africa and of respiratory syncytial virus (RSV) infection in infants in the United States. Its primary side effect has been a reversible suppression of hemoglobin production (hemoglobin is the protein that carries oxygen in the blood). Ribavirin treatment of cell cultures infected with HTLV-III/LAV indicates that the drug suppresses the virus with minimal damage to infected cells. Preliminary clinical trials are under way.

HPA-23 HPA-23 (antimoniotungstate) is a mineral compound discovered in France about 10 years ago. It inhibits reverse transcriptase activity of both mouse and human retroviruses. In preliminary clinical trials in France, the drug produced a decline in HTLV-III/LAV activity during therapy, but virus activity returned to pretreatment levels when therapy was stopped. Side effects include a temporary reduction in blood platelets (blood clotting cells) and reversible liver toxicity. Phase II trials of HPA-23 are under way in the United States and Europe.

Ansamycin The experimental drug ansamycin is being evaluated primarily in the treatment of *Mycobacterium avium-intracellulare* infections in AIDS patients (see Chapter 3), but recent evidence indicates that it also inhibits reverse transcriptase activity. The full implications of this finding are not yet known.

Cyclosporin A Cyclosporin A is a highly toxic immunosuppressive agent used to prevent rejection of organ transplants. It became the focus of extensive media attention in October 1985 after a group of French scientists announced that it had improved the immune status of two patients, one with AIDS and one with ARC, after only a week of therapy. The short study period and the small sample size led many researchers to question the validity of these findings. Some expressed concern that the drug would actually make AIDS patients more susceptible to infection, because it inhibits the same lymphocyte population attacked by HTLV-III/LAV. Patients who have received cyclosporin A following transplants and then developed transfusion-associated AIDS have fared very poorly. Further clinical trials of this drug are under way in Europe.

Immune Stimulators Early in the course of the AIDS epidemic, some scientists speculated that the most effective treatment for the severe immune defects associated with the syndrome might involve techniques to rebuild or stimulate the immune system. Researchers at the National Institute of Allergy and Infectious Diseases, for example, treated several AIDS patients with a combination of bone marrow transplants and lymphocyte transfers from their identical twin brothers. These efforts sometimes resulted in improved immunologic function, but the patients did not improve clinically, probably because the virus was still present. Additional studies are under way using bone marrow transplantation from an identical twin combined with antiviral therapy.

Other efforts to stimulate natural body defense mechanisms have involved use of the following: interleukin-2 (IL-2), an immune-system growth factor produced by T lymphocytes, the white blood cells most often attacked by HTLV-III/LAV; Isoprinosine, an immune-system modulator first created as a memory enhancer; hormones produced by the thymus gland; and gamma interferon, another protein derived from T lymphocytes. In early clinical trials, none of these substances used alone altered the deteriorating clinical condition of AIDS patients, probably because of the continuing viral infection. In fact, substances that stimulate the multiplication of T and B lymphocytes, such as IL-2, may simply create more target cells for replication of HTLV-III/LAV, resulting in more virus particles.

Combination Therapies   Although neither the current generation of antiviral drugs nor immunostimulatory techniques appear to alter the course of AIDS when used alone, scientists believe that combinations of the two might be effective. For example, an antiviral drug might be used with IL-2 therapy to protect healthy, dividing cells from the effects of the virus. Efforts to find the best combinations for different stages of disease will take time, however. Each combination therapy will have to undergo the same phases of clinical trials used to test single-drug regimens.

Another alternative is to combine antiviral drugs that act at different stages in the life cycle of HTLV-III/LAV. A substance that inhibits reverse transcriptase might be combined with interferon, for example. Alternating drugs might decrease the risk of side effects, an important goal if prolonged therapy is needed by millions of patients.

Designing New Drugs

The apparent failure of most known drugs to produce improvement in AIDS patients and the potential side effects of these agents have led some researchers to seek alternative strategies. Collaborative efforts by government and industry researchers have resulted in entirely new drugs capable of inhibiting HTLV-III/LAV in the laboratory. At least one of these substances, azidothymidine, also has shown promise in early clinical trials.

To identify potential antiviral agents, scientists use a screening system consisting of special T-lymphocyte cells that are unusually sensitive to destruction by HTLV-III/LAV. When virus particles alone are added to these cells in culture, all cells die within five or six days. Drug candidates are selected on the basis of their ability to protect the cells from the effects of the virus.

This system permits rapid testing of hundreds of agents. When a new substance is judged to be moderately effective, researchers explore ways to manipulate its chemical structure, hoping to find a variation that is even more potent than the original.

Azidothymidine, the first drug to make the transition from screening test to clinical trials, closely resembles one of the natural building blocks of DNA. Scientists believe that it inhibits replication of HTLV-III/LAV by taking the place of this essential building block during the conversion of viral RNA into DNA. When the viral enzyme reverse transcriptase mistakenly places azidothymidine in the DNA chain instead of the correct molecule, viral DNA formation stops. Reverse transcriptase appears much more likely to make this mistake than are enzymes that regulate the formation of cellular DNA, so therapeutic doses of azidothymidine do not appear to damage normal human cells.

Early clinical studies with azidothymidine have been very encouraging. Some AIDS patients treated with relatively low doses of the drug have shown rising T-cell counts and increases in absolute numbers of T4 lymphocytes. These and other changes in immune status have occurred after less than three weeks of therapy. Robert Yarchoan of the National Cancer Institute and his co-workers also have described short-term clinical improvements associated with azidothymidine therapy.

In addition to its apparent ability to improve immunologic function in AIDS patients, azidothymidine also satisfies other important criteria for a potential anti–HTLV-III/LAV drug, says Samuel Broder, director of the Clinical Oncology

Program at the National Cancer Institute. It is effective when given by mouth, and significant amounts cross the blood–brain barrier.

These results are very preliminary, but they indicate that a single agent may be able to suppress the virus and at the same time produce some regeneration of immune function. Azidothymidine will be one of the first agents tested in treatment evaluation units now being established around the country under the auspices of the National Institutes of Health.

An AIDS Vaccine

Public health education and the development of effective treatment strategies to suppress the virus are the principal short-term goals in the fight against AIDS, but the only hope for halting the spread of disease completely is widespread immunization. Scientists do not yet know how difficult it will be to produce a vaccine against HTLV-III/LAV. Even if a prototype is developed relatively quickly, the logistics of testing such a vaccine could add years to the time required for licensure in the United States.

Most familiar antiviral vaccines, including those for measles, mumps, and rubella, consist of live viruses that have been weakened (attenuated) in the laboratory so that they elicit a protective response without causing disease. Researchers generally believe that this strategy is not appropriate for HTLV-III/LAV because the virus is simply too dangerous. The possibility of an attenuated strain regaining its capacity to cause disease is too high.*

Several recent advances in molecular biology may offer alternative strategies. The most likely possibility is a subunit

---

*In March 1986, researchers at the Dana-Farber Cancer Institute and the National Cancer Institute announced simultaneously that they could produce intact but dead HTLV-III/LAV viruses by deleting the *tat*-III gene (see Chapter 4) from the viral genome. These genetically killed viruses look exactly like the complete virus, but they cannot reproduce. Researchers are exploring the feasibility of using genetically killed viruses in a vaccine; the safety of such a vaccine will depend on whether or not scientists can produce a defective virus that cannot become reactivated.

vaccine based on recombinant DNA technology. In this process, scientists identify the viral protein (antigen) most likely to arouse a protective antibody response from the human immune system. (This protein usually is part of the viral envelope, its outer coat.) The researchers pinpoint the portion of the viral genome coding for this protein, isolate it, and insert it into the genetic apparatus of another replicating virus, bacterium, yeast, or animal cell.

The outcome is a hybrid organism that replicates and produces the desired protein molecule in large quantities. Purification of the antigen results in a highly specific vaccine. Preliminary trials of a hepatitis B vaccine based on this strategy have been quite successful in humans. In addition, a subunit vaccine against feline leukemia virus (an animal retrovirus) is now available for immunization of kittens.

Certain characteristics of HTLV-III/LAV and its interactions with the human immune system complicate efforts to develop a potential subunit vaccine. The first is that the virus keeps changing its coat; it has an unusually high mutation rate, and the most variable segment of the genome is that coding for the envelope protein. Thus, antibodies generated against the envelope from one strain of HTLV-III/LAV might not recognize the envelope of another strain.

Some segments of the viral genome coding for the protein coat are less likely to change than others. This suggests that certain parts of the envelope protein may remain constant among different strains of HTLV-III/LAV. Many researchers believe, however, that these constant regions are hidden inside the protein molecule, out of reach of protective antibodies. Scientists are using complex biochemical techniques to dissect the envelope protein and to identify the best approach to this problem.

The second major barrier to the development of a vaccine is that scientists still are not sure that antibodies alone can protect the body against HTLV-III/LAV. Immunity to the virus may require a much more complex response involving many different functions of the immune system. Studies of AIDS patients and others infected with HTLV-III/LAV show that many do not make protective antibodies, and most of those who do make them have very low levels.

Clinical researchers are exploring the correlation between the presence of neutralizing antibodies and clinical disease. If infected persons who do not get sick are found to have higher levels of neutralizing antibody than those who succumb to opportunistic infections and other signs of AIDS, then prospects for a successful vaccine will be much brighter.

Perhaps the biggest advantage scientists have in the search for an AIDS vaccine is the existence of several animal models of the disease. Researchers in several laboratories have succeeded in infecting chimpanzees with HTLV-III/LAV. These animals do not develop the opportunistic infections or cancers characteristic of AIDS, but they do show immunologic changes and a predictable antibody response to the virus. Thus, they offer a valuable system in which to test prototype vaccines. (Unfortunately, such models generally are not suitable for testing the efficacy of potential therapeutic drugs.) The number of chimpanzees available for biomedical research is extremely limited, however, and so great care must be taken to ensure that vaccine tests are carefully planned and executed.

Myron Essex of the Harvard School of Public Health and his colleagues have isolated a retrovirus similar to HTLV-III/LAV—simian T-lymphotropic virus type III (STLV-III)—from both captive macaques with immune deficiency syndrome and healthy wild African green monkeys. The African green monkeys are particularly interesting because they seem to harbor the virus without getting sick. Scientists are not yet sure whether this resistance to disease occurs because the monkeys carry a weaker strain of retrovirus or because they have developed a more effective defense mechanism. Studies of interactions between STLV-III and the immune systems of these primates may lead to new strategies in the battle against human retroviral disease.

The importance of STLV-III was underscored recently by reports that blood samples from some healthy West African people contain antibodies against a virus that closely resembles the monkey retrovirus. If infection with the new virus proves to be protective against AIDS, then portions of its protein coat, or that of STLV-III, may be a logical choice for an AIDS vaccine.

Estimates of when a prototype vaccine might be available range from 1 year to 10 years or longer, depending on the outcome of current scientific studies. But even after a prototype is in hand, many years may pass before it is ready for widespread use. Testing of vaccines is extremely expensive and complex. The problems are compounded for a potential AIDS vaccine because of the long lag time between infection and the appearance of disease.

Clinical trials with such a vaccine will require thousands of willing, thoroughly informed research subjects who are at high risk but are still uninfected. After immunization they will have to be followed for years to detect signs of adverse reactions and to determine vaccine efficacy. The logistics of such a project will be massive, but attendant questions of liability may present even more of an impediment. Who will be willing to take responsibility for a vaccine when so much remains to be learned about how the virus attacks the body?

Another important need is to identify the ultimate target population for a vaccine. It cannot help those who are already infected, including the majority of American hemophiliacs and large portions of the male homosexual populations of major U.S. cities. Is the American public prepared for another attempt at mass immunization after the swine flu experience?

The problems of vaccine development discussed above are not insurmountable. Cooperative efforts between government and industry have accounted for extraordinary progress in other areas of AIDS research and may bring solutions to some of these problems. For the present, however, immunization should not be viewed as an imminent solution to the worldwide epidemic of HTLV-III/LAV-related diseases.

Conclusion

Education and other public health measures are the only tools now available to limit the spread of HTLV-III/LAV infection in the United States. Public health programs must continue to address the needs of high-risk groups and also must increase risk-reduction education for the general population.

Scientists have not yet developed effective strategies to treat HTLV-III/LAV infection, but several experimental programs have produced encouraging results. In addition to suppressing viral activity in the body, candidate drugs must be suitable for oral administration, must be able to cross the blood–brain barrier, and must be safe enough for lifelong use.

The prospects for a vaccine against HTLV-III/LAV appear less promising. In addition to the technical problems associated with initial development, the logistics and expense of clinical trials and associated liability issues present great obstacles. Mass immunization against AIDS should not be regarded as a reasonable option for the near future.

The most realistic goal now is to slow the spread of HTLV-III/LAV infection by employing a combination of health education and other public health measures. Policymakers in areas that have not been severely affected by the AIDS crisis should not wait to implement these programs, because the long latency period and the large number of infected persons without symptoms make it very difficult to assess the magnitude of the AIDS problem.

* * *

Chapter 6 is based on the presentations of Anthony S. Fauci, National Institute of Allergy and Infectious Diseases; James W. Curran, Centers for Disease Control; Mervyn F. Silverman, consultant and former Director of Health for San Francisco; Richard T. Johnson, Johns Hopkins University School of Medicine; Brett J. Cassens, American Association of Physicians for Human Rights; and June E. Osborn, School of Public Health, University of Michigan. Thanks also go to Jerome E. Groopman of the New England Deaconess Hospital and Martin S. Hirsch of Massachusetts General Hospital for their assistance in completing this chapter.

7

Individual and Societal Stress

The psychological and social effects of HTLV-III/LAV infection are as varied as the physical symptoms produced by the virus. Images of isolation and anguish experienced by patients and their families and friends blend into other images of fear and misunderstanding within their communities.

• A successful attorney loses his job and his closest friend less than a week after the doctor tells him he has Kaposi's sarcoma; his physician recommends a local AIDS support group, but when he enters the group's meeting room he is overwhelmed by the signs of advanced disease and flees.
• A middle-aged couple and their grown children sit on the edge of the living-room sofa, straining to hear the voice of the youngest son; they know that he is ill, but the revelation that he has AIDS leaves half of them in tears and the rest in stony silence.
• A man in a business suit paces up and down the hospital corridors trying to contain his anger and frustation; uncomfortable at his presence, family members of the man who has been his lover for more than five years have requested that he leave the patient's bedside.
• A young boy with hemophilia, barred from attending school because he has AIDS, sits alone in front of a blank television monitor waiting for the teacher at the other end of the closed-circuit hookup to begin the day's instruction.
• Infants in the nursery of a metropolitan hospital, vic-

tims of AIDS acquired in the womb, cry for mothers who do not come, either because they themselves are ill or because they cannot face the burden of caring for a child with such tremendous needs.

• The healthy older brother of a toddler with AIDS-related complex sits at the front of the classroom in a seat usually reserved for students who misbehave; teachers in his New Jersey school mistakenly believe that he could transmit the disease to his classmates.

• In New York City, frightened children march in picket lines carrying signs hand-lettered in crayon by their parents; the signs read "No Children with AIDS in Any of Our Grades" or "I Don't Want to Be the Next AIDS Victim."

• A city vehicle in San Antonio, Texas, pulls up to the curb at the home of a recently diagnosed AIDS patient; the official hand-delivers a letter warning the sick man that he faces felony charges if he engages in sexual intercourse with anyone other than another AIDS victim.

These scenes do not cover the full range of responses to the AIDS epidemic. They do not, for example, show the compassion and understanding of thousands of volunteers who provide emotional and practical support to AIDS patients across the nation, the dedication of health care personnel who choose to devote their careers to these patients, or the family members who discard lifelong prejudices to help loved ones cope with death. They do, however, illustrate the broad range of psychosocial issues affecting AIDS patients and their families, healthy members of high-risk groups, and the general population.

AIDS Patients

The psychological impact of a diagnosis of AIDS is similar in some respects to that elicited by diagnoses of other fatal illnesses. The first response is often denial—in some cases so strong that patients refuse medical care. For most, however, the denial is tempered by realism. The result may be behaviors that seem contradictory, such as arranging to meet with a lawyer but refusing to sign a will. Whatever their initial reactions, AIDS patients need immediate and continuous access to counseling and a compassionate and understanding health care team.

The patient's response to AIDS depends in part on his or her psychological condition before the appearance of the syndrome. Patients with a history of psychiatric disorders are less likely than others to adjust to their illness and imminent death. Their inability to cope may become particularly evident when the physician recommends risk-reduction measures such as avoidance of sexual behaviors that could transmit the virus, reduced alcohol consumption, or elimination of drug abuse. In some cases, these proscribed behaviors may be the patient's principal ways of handling stress.

After the initial period of denial, most patients pass through a period characterized by alternating episodes of anger and depression, combined with fear about the future course of the disease and the effects of therapy. The anger may be especially severe in AIDS patients because of their relative youth. (Ninety percent of adults with the syndrome are between the ages of 20 and 49.) Death is difficult to face at any age, but a premature death often seems especially unfair. The fear may be exacerbated by recent experiences involving friends or acquaintances who succumbed to AIDS. Indeed, many patients have lost an entire social network to AIDS and are left without support for some of the most difficult months of their lives.

Health care professionals can help AIDS patients through these turbulent times by encouraging them to express their fears, providing accurate information, directing anger into constructive pathways (such as volunteer activities), prescribing appropriate medications (ranging from mild antianxiety drugs to stronger antidepressants, depending on the needs of the patient), and encouraging the development of new social contacts.

Eventually, the majority of AIDS patients who are not overwhelmed by neurological problems begin to accept the limitations of the disease and assume an active role in decisions about their future health care. Those who remain mobile often use the time to work at AIDS crisis centers or to participate in other community projects. As the disease progresses, the focus gradually shifts to preparations for death.

Several factors may make AIDS patients psychologically more vulnerable than people with other fatal illnesses. Some of these obstacles result from social issues, and others arise because of the nature of the virus.

Discrimination

The distribution of AIDS cases in the United States— more than 70 percent among homosexuals and 17 percent among intravenous drug abusers—has fostered the belief in some segments of society that AIDS is a form of punishment for socially unacceptable behavior. One AIDS patient recalls that his sister's first response upon hearing he had AIDS was: "You should be ashamed of yourself."

The concept of a "gay disease" has been extremely hard to change, despite knowledge that the syndrome is a viral illness transmitted by heterosexual as well as homosexual intercourse. The social stigma attached to the syndrome may be especially overwhelming for homosexual or bisexual men who have hidden their sexual orientation for years from family and friends. A few commit suicide rather than risk the rejection they expect when others become aware of their disease.

Homosexual men who have internalized society's disapproval of their sexual orientation may accept discrimination from others without complaint. Such discrimination can take various forms. Some patients with AIDS have lost both their jobs and their homes within weeks of the diagnosis, although these actions increasingly are being challenged in court. An employer or landlord who goes to great lengths to help a person with cancer or heart disease may be unwilling to exhibit the same compassion for an AIDS victim.

For AIDS patients, the trauma of being fired or evicted

quickly becomes subordinate to practical concerns about how and where they will live the last months of their lives. Many need immediate legal and financial counseling, as well as more conventional services. The comprehensive network of AIDS-related agencies in San Francisco provides a model for other regions preparing to deal with the psychosocial effects of the AIDS crisis. Working together, these agencies offer emergency housing and food services, free legal advice, practical support for daily living, substance abuse counseling, and extended home nursing care, as well as individual counseling for patients and their families. These accomplishments represent a cooperative effort by the local government and the San Francisco homosexual community.

In areas where the population of AIDS patients is more varied, the task of helping individuals and families deal with the social impact of the syndrome may be more difficult. Health care institutions in New York City have established special units to care for families in which one or both parents have AIDS or ARC as a result of drug abuse, but much more needs to be accomplished in this realm.

The problem of discrimination is not limited to homosexuals. Healthy siblings of children with transfusion-associated AIDS have been barred from nursery schools and day care centers. Court cases in several states attest to the discrimination faced by hemophiliacs with the syndrome. Televised lessons and private tutoring have been offered as alternatives to attending school for these children, but neither can be expected to satisfy the social or psychological needs of a third-grader or a young adolescent.

The plight of infants with AIDS may be especially desperate. Fear of contagion may deny them the cuddling and close contact essential for even a very short life.

Physical Limitations

Two characteristics of infection with HTLV-III/LAV also interfere with patients' efforts to cope with AIDS. The first is the many different clinical signs and symptoms associated with disruption of the immune system. A man with Kaposi's sarcoma may learn to accept the disfigurement of this cancer and adapt to cancer therapy, but when he suddenly develops *Pneumocystis carinii* pneumonia, his resiliency disappears. Each new manifestation of disease may elicit the same anger and fear associated with the original diagnosis and require a new period of adjustment.

The second problem, which is potentially much more serious, is the effect of HTLV-III/LAV on the brain. Brain disease caused by the virus may lead to gradual deterioration of mental faculties over a period of months. Health care providers must learn to watch for this process, which can affect the patient's ability to cope with the illness in a variety of ways.

In some cases mild memory loss or an inability to accomplish simple tasks may cause depression; in other cases the depression itself may be a symptom of the infection. Subtle personality changes may alter the way the patient relates to medical and nursing staff or result in an inability to comply with therapeutic regimens.

When dementia resulting from HTLV-III/LAV infection becomes more severe, the patient may be unable to participate in decisions about future care. One aspect of this problem is determining when an individual is capable of giving informed consent for an experimental procedure. Because medical science has had so little experience with AIDS, all drug regimens used to treat HTLV-III/LAV infection are experimental. A related concern is that some of these powerful agents also affect the central nervous system.

Researchers are developing a battery of neuropsychological and behavioral tests to assist physicians in differentiating between central nervous system disorders caused by the AIDS virus and stress-related psychological problems.

ARC Patients

Patients with AIDS-related complex (ARC) face many of the same stress factors as those with AIDS: physical limita-

tions, social prejudice, potential loss of economic self-suffi-
ciency, and the need to change high-risk behaviors. In fact, a
comparison of ARC and AIDS patients by Susan Tross and
Jimmie Holland at Memorial Sloan-Kettering Cancer Center
in New York City found that ARC patients exhibited a higher
level of social and psychological distress than AIDS patients.

This more intense reaction results primarily from the
uncertainty associated with ARC. Patients continually ask
themselves and others, "Will I be among the ARC patients
who develop AIDS?" They may become intensely angry with
health care providers who cannot answer this question.

ARC patients who feel well enough to continue participating in social activities also may have more difficulty adapt-
ing to risk-reduction behaviors than AIDS patients. Change
itself may become a focus of stress.

All patients with ARC require regular medical care, but
some have much greater needs than others. The symptoms of
ARC vary in severity from moderately painful swollen glands
to debilitating fevers and persistent diarrhea. Those with more
severe symptoms may be too weak to work or even to care for
themselves at home, yet they may be denied the financial and
social service benefits accorded to AIDS patients.

The psychological and social needs of these vulnerable
patients require further study to ensure that they receive the
range of services they need.

High-Risk But Healthy Individuals

Imagine the psychological impact of watching a dozen
friends under the age of 45 succumb to a fatal illness. For tens
of thousands of homosexual men in the United States, the
death of loved ones and friends has become a regular occurrence. For most of these men, the stress of constant grief has
been amplified by fear—fear that the next cough or skin
blemish will signal the beginning of their own battle with
AIDS.

AIDS has changed homosexual practices in this country
faster than anyone would have believed possible. It is almost as

if a film documenting the sexual revolution of the 1960s had been played backward at top speed. Studies throughout the country show a decrease in anonymous sexual encounters and other high-risk behaviors.

Homosexual communities have responded to the AIDS crisis by creating social and political organizations to aid the sick and to lobby for financial support of research and treatment facilities. Many of the men involved in these organizations had not publicly identified themselves as homosexuals before the crisis began—thus, these communities may be stronger and more unified than ever before. But anxiety levels are high. Conversations about AIDS have become a part of every social gathering. Some men develop physical symptoms that mimic those of HTLV-III/LAV infection. Others make frequent trips to the doctor seeking unrealistic guarantees.

The desire to know one's antibody status may conflict with fears of personal exposure should the results become known. Brett J. Cassens, former president of the American Association of Physicians for Human Rights (AAPHR), says that confidentiality "is considered by most gay persons to be the most important if not the only true defense against social discrimination."

Confidentiality with respect to AIDS testing and research is an extremely complex issue. As noted in Chapter 6, one state now requires laboratories to report to state health authorities the names and addresses of persons who have a confirmed positive HTLV-III/LAV antibody test. Despite assurances that this information will be handled with strict confidentiality, opponents of mandatory reporting are wary of any regulation that will establish a list of persons at high risk for AIDS. After all, half of the states in this country still have so-called sodomy laws, which make homosexual practices of any kind illegal.

In some areas, state and local health departments have worked with organizations within the homosexual community to design systems that offer the benefits of testing without subjecting those tested to the risk of disclosure. For example, a network linking alternative testing sites in Massachusetts uses a system in which anonymous clients call a central telephone number to receive an identification code and an appointment at the most convenient site. Counseling is provided before the test to ensure that each client understands the full significance of both positive and negative results.

To limit the spread of disease without resorting to the antibody test, the AAPHR recommends that all homosexual men assume that they are antibody-positive and behave accordingly (practice "safe sex" and good general health measures). June E. Osborn, dean of the School of Public Health at the University of Michigan, argues that these recommendations do not have the same effect as concrete information. She says that the difference between being instructed to assume that one is infected with HTLV-III/LAV and learning of a positive antibody test is like the difference between reading the literature on smoking and lung cancer and being told that a laboratory test has revealed abnormal cells in the lung. In both cases, she believes, test results are more likely to bring about risk-reduction behavior than is general information. Very little research has been done on the impact of different forms of health education.

Confidentiality issues also must be resolved to ensure the continued cooperation of high-risk groups in AIDS research. One of the most urgent needs in the battle against AIDS is to identify cofactors that increase the likelihood of infection with HTLV-III/LAV or that make infected individuals more likely to get sick (possible examples include other viruses, stress, and the use of recreational drugs). Knowledge of these cofactors could lead to new preventive techniques, but the only way to acquire the information needed is through long-term studies of high-risk volunteers.

Other research topics will require both high- and low-risk subjects. For example, studies of the factors that influence changes in sexual behavior should focus on both homosexuals and heterosexuals, with single and multiple partners. Data from such studies will be essential to increasing the effectiveness of public education materials.

Another important research goal is to learn more about the psychological impact of a positive test result on someone who is otherwise healthy. The needs of these high-risk individuals vary greatly: some may require intensive counseling to deal with the increased risk of disease and early death, while others may obtain sufficient support from regular visits to their physicians.

The General Population

Media polls in 1985 indicated that most adults in the United States were concerned but not panic-stricken about AIDS. School boycotts (protesting the attendance of children with AIDS in elementary schools) and job discrimination against those believed to belong to high-risk groups have been the exception rather than the rule. Frequent reassurances from the Centers for Disease Control have contributed to this relative calm, as have the broad changes in cultural and social attitudes toward homosexuals that originated two decades ago. But perhaps the most important explanation for the public's behavior to date has been the relatively low incidence of disease.

As the number of cases increases nationwide, however, pressures are increasing for more restrictive public health measures. Already, advocates of mandatory testing and similar public health measures have begun to attract new supporters. AIDS hotlines in major cities report that up to 75 percent of their calls now come from individuals who do not belong to high-risk groups. Perception of risk plays a major role in the public's willingness to listen to reassurances based on complex scientific data.

In some cases, lack of unanimity within the medical community has adversely affected public understanding of AIDS risk factors. Confusion is not surprising when physicians who lack knowledge about the syndrome air their own fears in an open forum. For example, in mid-1985 three physicians in a major southwestern city stood before the city council and warned members of their community to stop shaking hands with strangers because they might catch AIDS from sweaty palms. This advice probably had much more impact locally than did published statements by CDC epidemiologists.

Different interpretations of available data also cause confusion. This is inevitable when a new disease is the focus of constant media attention, but researchers should be aware of the consequences of their statements. Conflicting comments about the reliability of the AIDS antibody test and about the possibility of female-to-male transmission of the virus have been particularly widespread. The general public may conclude that if scientists cannot agree on these basic issues, perhaps they really do not know how the virus spreads.

Another source of communication difficulties is the conflict between the public's desire to hear definite "yes" or "no" answers and scientists' unwillingness to make absolute statements. This problem results in part from the nature of scientific training, but the major problem is the medical profession's lack of experience with this very new and complex syndrome.

The next few years will be crucial to efforts to slow the spread of HTLV-III/LAV infection. Widespread education about risk factors and the feasibility of different public health measures should begin now, while the audience is still receptive. Prompt action could forestall hysteria over a problem that will continue to be part of American society for the foreseeable future.

Health Care Personnel

Caring for patients with AIDS and other conditions caused by HTLV-III/LAV infection may be particularly draining for health care personnel. Watching the rapid deterioration and death of men and women who should be in the prime of life requires extraordinary emotional stamina, especially for those accustomed to winning medical battles against an array of lesser pathogens.

AIDS also may be emotionally threatening to health care personnel for other reasons. Despite numerous reports indicating that HTLV-III/LAV is not transmitted from patients to health care workers (except in very rare cases involving needle-stick injuries or similar accidents) some individuals may not be able to overcome fears about the possibility of infection. This may lead to inappropriate behavior, such as wearing more protective clothing than is necessary when caring for AIDS patients. (See Appendix B for PHS recommendations for preventing transmission of HTLV-III/LAV in health care settings.)

Frequent staff meetings at which workers feel comfortable expressing their concerns about personal safety and patient interactions are essential for any institution providing regular services for AIDS patients. These meetings also can provide a forum for continuing discussions about requirements for staffing. Most AIDS patients require very intensive care over long periods. The San Francisco experience suggests that one way to provide comprehensive care without overtaxing the medical system is to get help from volunteers. This approach may be less effective, however, in areas where the population of AIDS victims includes a mixture of persons from different high-risk groups.

Some physicians, nurses, and support staff may be unable to work effectively with AIDS patients because of prejudices against homosexuality or intravenous drug abusers. For example, if a physician feels uncomfortable discussing sexuality issues with a homosexual patient or believes that any attempt to educate drug abusers about health risks is a waste of time, then that physician cannot offer the comprehensive care needed by such patients. These attitudes must be addressed openly. Because they are unlikely to change over time, the best solution may be to reassign the individual to another part of the health care facility.

Conclusion

The psychosocial impact of HTLV-III/LAV infection should not be underestimated. AIDS transforms the lives of patients, their families, and friends, but its effects are not limited to high-risk groups. Fear of the syndrome, its devastating complications and high mortality rate, is increasing. Much of this fear is based on erroneous information, but public reactions should not be discounted as mass hysteria. The epidemic is real and policymakers must do everything possible to promote a realistic approach to this complex problem.

For now, prevention through risk-reduction education and other public health measures is the only effective weapon against this disease. Data on homosexual groups indicate that behavioral change is possible with appropriate educational materials, but researchers still know very little about whether these changes will last or about how to reach other segments of society. Studies of the factors that influence sexual behavior and drug abuse among both high- and low-risk groups should be given high priority.

Psychosocial factors also may play a role in determining a person's susceptibility to infection or susceptibility to disease once the virus has entered the body. For example, scientists in other fields have shown a direct link between stress and immune function. If stress is shown to be a cofactor in the development of AIDS-related opportunistic infections, then stress-reduction techniques could save lives. Researchers at the National Institute of Mental Health and other organizations have begun long-term studies of high-risk subjects to determine the relationship between psychological status and immunological and clinical function.

Efforts to plan for the future health care needs of patients infected with HTLV-III/LAV also depend on greater knowledge about the range of neuropsychiatric problems caused by the virus. The prevalence of mild to severe dementia among AIDS victims may be much higher than previously suspected. Clinicians need better tests to monitor changes in mental function. Without these tests, it may be very difficult to assess the patient's capabilities with respect to self-care and compliance with therapeutic regimens. Unrealistic expectations in these areas could be a source of extreme frustration for both the patient and the medical staff.

The majority of AIDS cases in the United States have

been concentrated in urban centers in New York, California, Florida, New Jersey, the District of Columbia, and Texas, but there is evidence that over the next two or three years other parts of the country will become more heavily burdened. These new patients and the communities in which they live will require knowledgeable physicians, nurses, dentists, psychologists, social workers, and a vast array of support services. Education of these professionals, encompassing both the psychosocial and the health effects of the syndrome, should be given high priority by educational institutions, professional societies, and the government.

* * *

Chapter 7 is based on the presentations of Shervert Frazier, National Institute of Mental Health; Brett J. Cassens, American Association of Physicians for Human Rights; and Ronald Bayer, The Hastings Center.

8

Public Health Policy

If a panel of public health experts, lawyers, economists, and sociologists had been asked a decade ago to imagine a public health problem that would encompass the most difficult policy issues of the day, they could not have done better than predict the appearance of AIDS. The AIDS epidemic raises basic questions about the rights of individuals versus those of society, about the government's role in the provision of health care, and about the manner in which our social structure responds to new challenges.

Initial efforts to develop consistent policies with regard to AIDS were hampered by lack of knowledge about the syndrome. For the first two to three years of the epidemic, society battled an unknown enemy. This lack of information was frightening, but it also allowed policymakers to maintain an optimistic outlook: surely, once biomedical researchers had identified the cause of AIDS, treatments and vaccines would follow and the social problems associated with the syndrome would disappear.

Despite remarkable scientific advances, HTLV-III/LAV has proved to be an extremely tough opponent. It rapidly integrates itself into the genetic machinery of human target cells. Although several drugs appear to inhibit replication of the virus, none has produced clinical improvement in AIDS patients. Other characteristics of the virus, discussed in detail earlier, complicate efforts to develop a vaccine.

A further complexity is posed by the fact that the

infection has an unusually long latency period. Public health planning is very difficult when no one knows how many of those carrying the infection will eventually develop full-blown AIDS. Moreover, scientists now recognize that AIDS is only one possible outcome of HTLV-III/LAV infection; the virus also causes debilitating brain disease and may precipitate a range of cancers and infections not included in the Centers for Disease Control's definition of the syndrome. Many years will pass before researchers know what proportion of those infected with the virus will be able to resist its effects and live normal lives.

Another characteristic of the virus that has had a major impact on the development of public health strategies has been the unexpected finding that most of those who have antibodies against the virus also carry active virus particles. This means that the pool of potentially infectious persons is not limited to AIDS and ARC patients; in fact, the estimated million or more persons who carry the virus but have no symptoms may be more infectious than those with the full-blown disease.

Concern over the potential for discrimination against the groups most affected by the syndrome, especially homosexuals, also has had a significant impact on AIDS policies. Prejudice against homosexuals has played a role in housing and employment problems encountered by individual AIDS victims and has affected the quality of health care in some cases.

Leaders of homosexual organizations have been particularly concerned about the ability of AIDS researchers to protect the privacy of the thousands of research subjects (many of whom are healthy, but antibody-positive, members of high-risk groups) who have volunteered to participate in studies of the natural history of HTLV-III/LAV infection. Representatives of these organizations have worked closely with government researchers to ensure that guarantees of confidentiality are explicit and that the identities of research subjects cannot be obtained by anyone who might use them for discriminatory purposes.

Another aspect of this issue is the government's fear of

appearing discriminatory. Because such a large proportion of AIDS victims are homosexuals, it is very difficult to design preventive measures that do not have the appearance of discriminating against them.

Funding decisions also have been scrutinized for evidence of discrimination. About half of American adults polled in September 1985 by ABC News and the *Washington Post* believed that the U.S. government would have spent more on AIDS research if the disease had not mainly affected homosexual men.

The Costs of Fighting AIDS

Estimates of the cost of hospital care for a single AIDS patient range from $42,000 to $147,000.* The projected cost of AIDS-related health care in New York City for 1986 is between $110 million and $150 million. The federal government spent $109 million on AIDS research and education in 1985, and is expected to spend about $200 million in 1986.

The economic impact of the epidemic will continue to grow as the disease spreads. The increase in number of cases will have a disproportionate impact on the demand for health care resources because a much higher proportion of patients will be using health care facilities at the same time. This effect will be magnified if early therapeutic techniques prolong lives without producing significant improvements in health status.

AIDS can no longer be regarded as a local problem for a few major cities with large patient populations. The syndrome has now been reported in all 50 states. Policymakers at every level of government, business leaders, and members of the general public must confront the economic challenges pre-

---

*The estimate of $147,000 for the amount expended for the hospital care of each AIDS patient was reported by CDC researcher Ann M. Hardy and her colleagues in the *Journal of the American Medical Association*, Jan. 10, 1986. The authors acknowledge that this estimate may be high, "in part, because data on hospitalization after initial stay were available only from New York City, and hospital use by patients with AIDS there may be greater than by patients in other areas" (p. 210).

sented by the epidemic and help develop creative new approaches to meet them.

Funding decisions at the federal level focus on how much money should be allocated to AIDS—and on what other diseases will lose funding because of it; on the appropriate balance between basic biomedical research and other types of research; on how to fund and structure risk-reduction education and clinical drug trials; and on whether the federal government should become involved directly in patient care. For state and local governments, the principal funding issue is how to help patients and health care facilities cope with the tremendous financial burdens imposed by AIDS and related diseases (California, New York, and several other states also fund AIDS research).*

The Federal Government's Response

The federal government's response to AIDS has been marked by a tug of war between the administration and Congress. A technical memorandum produced by the Congress's Office of Technology Assessment described this process in February 1985:

> Through the Assistant Secretary for Health, individual PHS [Public Health Service] agencies have consistently asked DHHS [the Department of Health and Human Services] to request particular sums from Congress; the Department has submitted requests for amounts smaller than those suggested by the agencies; and Congress typically has appropriated amounts greater than those requested by the Department.†

---

*State and local governments have varied in their approaches to the AIDS problem. For specific information on individual states, consult *A Review of State and Local Government Initiatives Affecting AIDS* (November 1985), prepared by the Intergovernmental Health Policy Project at the George Washington University, with the assistance of the Association of State and Territorial Health Officials, the National Governors' Association, and the U.S. Conference of Mayors.

†"Review of the Public Health Service's Response to AIDS. A Technical Memorandum," OTA-TM-H-24 (Washington, D.C.: U.S. Congress, Office of Technology Assessment), p. 7.

The budgetary process for 1986 provides a good example. The administration's initial budget request for AIDS research for 1986 was $85.6 million, later raised to $126.3 million. In response, Congress appropriated $244 million. The Office of Management and Budget countered by including a proposal to cancel about 20 percent of this amount in its draft budget for 1987, which called for $193 million for AIDS research for 1986 and $213 million for 1987. (These figures probably will continue to change as the budgetary process continues.)

Several factors account for this dispute. Certainly, concern over the federal budget deficit has cast a long shadow over a wide range of issues, including AIDS spending. In addition, the emergence of the AIDS epidemic has coincided with a trend toward reduced federal involvement in all types of domestic social programs.

The rapid evolution of the AIDS crisis also has contributed to uncertainty over funding levels. Budgetary mechanisms are not designed to deal with problems that change from day to day. Thus, much of the funding for AIDS has had to come through supplemental requests and reprogramming of existing funds. This has created considerable competition among Public Health Service agencies involved in fighting the disease.

The largest proportion of the federal AIDS budget has been devoted to basic biomedical research. Much of what is now known about the natural history of HTLV-III/LAV infection has resulted from these federally sponsored activities. Some observers have expressed concern, however, that the government has not devoted sufficient resources to prevention, to behavioral research, or to the development of new therapeutic techniques.

Prevention through risk-reduction education and other public health measures is currently the only way to slow the spread of AIDS. Federal budget requests reflect growing recognition of this fact: the 1986 budget includes more than $20 million for the education of both high- and low-risk groups. Most of these funds will be distributed through the Centers for Disease Control to state and local organizations.

AIDS-prevention education would gain a new dimension if scientists could identify factors that alter the risk of disease for those already infected with HTLV-III/LAV. Potential cofactors include other medical problems and psychosocial risk factors such as stress, exhaustion, anxiety, and the loss of social support. Cofactor research requires long-term follow-up of thousands of high-risk volunteers; funding in this area has increased over time, but perhaps not in proportion to its potential impact.

Federal procedures and funding for the development of new anti-AIDS drugs came under sharp attack in mid-1985, following reports that many American AIDS patients were seeking treatment outside the United States. Scientists in this country responded to this criticism by noting that clinical trials would have been meaningless before the discovery of HTLV-III/LAV and the development of reliable laboratory tests.

Funding for research on therapeutic agents has increased substantially since the identification of the virus. The National Institutes of Health (NIH) has established a drug evaluation committee to identify promising agents and to make recommendations about initiating clinical trials. This committee works closely with the Food and Drug Administration to ensure that the process moves as rapidly as possible. In addition, the National Institute of Allergy and Infectious Diseases is organizing a nationwide network of medical centers to conduct phase II clinical trials of promising drugs. All of these efforts are designed to ensure that no information is wasted; each clinical trial will build on information accumulated in previous trials. The result will be precise knowledge about the safety and efficacy of a wide range of potential treatment alternatives.

Despite these cooperative efforts, some observers believe there is a need for a central office to plan and coordinate federally sponsored AIDS-related programs. The responsibilities of such an office would include improving communication among researchers and minimizing the adverse effects of competition for limited funds. The House Appropriations Committee has recommended that a permanent AIDS chief be appointed within the Department of Health and Human Services. Others have suggested the creation of a new institute within NIH to deal specifically with AIDS. The Institute of Medicine (IOM) jointly with the National Academy of Sciences (NAS) is examining these and other options in a major effort to develop a national research and health care agenda for AIDS.

Major questions remain about the best way to implement this agenda once it has been established. Most current research on HTLV-III/LAV is concentrated in a few government, industry, and academic laboratories. The involvement of more researchers might increase the speed at which new ideas are evaluated and incorporated into clinical practice. Another concern is the appropriate balance between government- and industry-funded research. Commercial involvement in the fight against AIDS is crucial, but policymakers must address the inherent conflict between the proprietary rights of individual firms and the need for open communication.

Organizing and Financing Clinical Services

The IOM/NAS committee also will explore the difficult problem of how to organize and finance clinical and supportive services for AIDS patients. A sudden influx of AIDS patients can throw a single hospital department or an entire medical center into disarray. Hospitals need to develop specific plans that will allow them to provide comprehensive care for AIDS patients without disrupting other services. Community-wide efforts are needed to ensure that individual institutions are not overburdened; the needs of both patients and staff must be considered in planning an equitable distribution of cases.

The estimated costs of hospitalization for each AIDS patient—from $42,000 to $147,000—are now being met through a combination of sources: private health insurance, direct out-of-pocket payments by patients, Medicare, Medicaid, and other state and local funds. Increasingly, however, insurance companies are seeking ways to avoid covering those who might develop AIDS, and public hospitals are finding that they can no longer cope with this enormous drain on their resources. In addition, many public and private insurers pay only for established and standard treatments, while the most promising treatments for AIDS and related conditions are still experimental.

As the number of AIDS cases increases nationwide, these problems will worsen. In some areas, the fastest-growing segment of the AIDS population consists of intravenous drug abusers. These individuals are more likely to be indigent than earlier AIDS patients were, and they often require a greater range of services.

Evidence from San Francisco suggests that community-based programs, including home nursing care and hospice services, may reduce the cost of AIDS and at the same time provide a more humane environment for AIDS patients. However, these alternative health care delivery systems require a strong commitment from local organizations, a commitment that may not exist in some parts of the country.

Decisions about how to pay for the high cost of AIDS may have profound implications for the future of health care financing in general in this country. Many of the problems generated by the AIDS crisis are comparable to those created by other catastrophic illnesses, such as cancer. Thus, effective methods of dealing with the AIDS crisis could be used as a model for developing a more coherent approach to an entire range of related funding issues. This makes it vitally important that every segment of society take an active role in these decisions.

Balancing Health Needs and Individual Rights

Managing the financial burdens associated with AIDS is just one aspect of the very complex public health dilemma presented by the syndrome. An equally difficult problem, common to any effort to control an epidemic, is how to balance the health needs of the community against the individual civil rights of those capable of transmitting the disease.

As noted in Chapter 6, public health measures consist of

a range of options including general education, specific education for high-risk groups, voluntary testing and counseling, mandatory reporting of test results, contact tracing, regulations to close establishments associated with high-risk behavior, mandatory testing, and various forms of quarantine. Public health officials have the very difficult task of deciding whether compelling state interests require movement from voluntary measures to the more restrictive end of this spectrum. Needless to say, each step in this progression occasions considerable public discussion.

In most areas, efforts to limit the transmission of HTLV-III/LAV involve only education and voluntary testing and counseling, but more restrictive measures have been adopted in certain situations. The following section describes three of these situations: (1) actions by San Francisco and New York authorities to restrict certain activities associated with increased risk for the transmission of HTLV-III/LAV (which ultimately resulted in the closing of establishments that encourage or facilitate multiple anonymous sexual encounters among homosexuals); (2) a decision by a Florida judge to put a female prostitute with AIDS under house arrest to prevent her from transmitting the disease to others; and (3) a directive by the Department of Defense to test 2.1 million active and reserve servicemen for HTLV-III/LAV antibodies.

Mervyn F. Silverman, former Director of Health for San Francisco, explains that his ruling to close gay bathhouses and sex clubs in that city was an agonizing decision that evolved over many months. Initially, health officials had hoped that educational efforts to change sexual behaviors throughout the homosexual community would obviate the need for restrictive measures of any kind. (In fact, they were concerned that restrictive measures might reduce the level of cooperation.) They also believed that by placing educational materials in the bathhouses, they might influence a segment of the homosexual population that otherwise would have been extremely difficult to reach.

It soon became clear, however, that the owners of these establishments were ignoring the risk of AIDS, Silverman says. They were profiting from high-risk behaviors at the same time that the city was spending millions of dollars to control transmission of the syndrome. In August 1984 Silverman ordered the businesses closed.

No one expected that closing the bathhouses would stop the spread of AIDS, but the San Francisco authorities believed that the city could not continue to give tacit approval to businesses that actively encouraged such dangerous activities. Silverman explains that operation of the bathhouses presented a direct challenge to community standards about the value of life—the same type of challenge that would be presented by an entrepreneur who sought permission to open an inviting, softly lit Russian roulette parlor.

Reactions among homosexuals to the decision in San Francisco and to similar actions by the State Public Health Council of New York have been mixed. Some of those opposed to such measures have said that public health officials do not have enough data about the risks presented by these establishments to justify closing them. Others worry that these rulings could establish dangerous precedents for further restrictive measures against homosexuals, including the reinstitution of sodomy laws. The civil liberties issues are extremely complex. Does the government have the right to close establishments primarily to curtail interactions between consenting adults or are such actions a violation of the constitutional right to privacy? When do the rights of individuals become subordinate to those of society as a whole?

Concern over individual rights looms larger as communities across the country seek to reactivate local quarantine laws. Before the development of antibiotics and other wonders of modern medicine, these laws were important tools in the battle against infectious disease. Many older citizens still remember the boldly lettered signs that indicated the presence of diphtheria or whooping cough in a household.

Unlike these other diseases, however, AIDS is not thought to be transmitted through casual contact; the types of behavior that spread the syndrome are well understood. AIDS patients and others who know they are infected with HTLV-III/LAV and who comply with public health guidelines regarding transmission of the virus present no danger to the community.

Spokesmen for some religious and political groups have asked public health officials why they do not simply quarantine all those capable of spreading the disease. Such an act would be totally unnecessary and unjustified, as well as impractical. It would mean quarantining more than a million people for life.

The most likely use of quarantine laws in the control of AIDS would be to restrict the activities of those who continue high-risk behaviors without regard for the health of others. This issue has arisen primarily with respect to HTLV-III/LAV-infected prostitutes—men and women who refuse to leave the streets. In one case, a Florida judge confined a female prostitute with AIDS to her home and enforced the order by requiring her to wear an electronic bracelet that would alert police if she strayed too far from the monitoring device placed in her telephone.

The use of quarantine laws to slow the spread of AIDS raises many ethical, moral, and legal questions. For example, at what point should educational efforts give way to restrictive measures such as house arrest? Does society have a responsibility to provide for those who are confined as a result of quarantine laws? What is society's responsibility to those who engage in sexual intercourse with prostitutes?

Some public health officials worry that even very limited use of quarantine laws might dissuade AIDS victims from seeking therapy or from participating in crucial clinical research programs. The benefits of preventing one person from spreading the disease might be outweighed by losing contact with many more individuals who would respond to educational efforts.

Perhaps the best illustration of the complexity of establishing policies to deal with the AIDS crisis is the situation in the U.S. military. Blood tests have been used to screen out new recruits with HTLV-III/LAV antibodies since the fall of 1985, and efforts are now under way to test all men and women on active duty.

Military sources state that these actions are necessary to ensure the continued strength of the armed forces; to ensure that personnel in combat areas are available to provide transfusions for an injured comrade without the risk of transmitting AIDS; to protect the health of those whose natural defense mechanisms have been compromised by infection with HTLV-III/LAV; and to protect the sexual partners of military personnel in other countries. They note that recruits with weakened immune systems might have severe adverse reactions to the numerous immunizations required for military service. In addition, military personnel who carry the virus might be more susceptible to tropical diseases encountered during overseas assignments.

The decision to initiate widespread screening led to general confusion within the military services about what should be done with regard to those who test positive. The activities most often associated with transmission of the virus—homosexuality and drug abuse—are considered grounds for dismissal without benefits by all branches of the military. Department of Defense guidelines make it clear, however, that the services cannot use a positive HTLV-III/LAV antibody test result as a basis for deciding that an individual has engaged in these activities (although they do not prohibit investigation of the possible cause of the presence of the antibodies).

In general, the services have decided that persons who test positive and have signs of disease will be processed for medical disability. Those who have evidence of exposure but appear clinically normal will be retained in the military, although with possible assignment limitations (including no overseas duty). Individual rulings could be affected, however, by evidence of misconduct (that is, homosexuality or drug abuse) independent of the medical evaluation.

Spokesmen for homosexuals have criticized the military screening program on several grounds. They believe that the underlying purpose of testing for exposure to HTLV-III/LAV is to identify homosexuals in the armed forces, and that the decision barring recruits who test positive but are otherwise healthy is designed primarily to avoid the costs of caring for these individuals if they should become sick. The provision for limited duty has been viewed as a threat to career advancement for individuals who had planned to spend their entire adult lives in the military.

A more general concern, however, is that the military's decision will encourage other large organizations to implement similar screening programs. Employers throughout the country have begun to consider screening, and insurance companies are seeking permission to test applicants for new policies. Several states are investigating the possibility of testing their prison populations.

Society must decide whether the health needs of the community justify the infringements on civil liberties associated with such measures. Decisions of this type will arise with greater frequency if educational programs fail to effect widespread behavioral changes.

The AIDS crisis sheds light on the ways in which social mores affect our ability to cope with new problems. For example, in October 1985, the Los Angeles City Council refused to allow the city health department to put out a flyer on AIDS and drug abuse because the councillors felt that it reflected a permissive attitude toward drug use. (The flyer stated that drug abuse was a problem for many reasons, but that those who used drugs anyway should at least make sure their equipment was clean.) City, state, and federal authorities also have hesitated to support the distribution of explicit risk-reduction education materials for homosexuals.

These actions reflect the views that government institutions should not be telling people how to conduct illegal activities and that some topics are not appropriate for public discussion. Health experts argue that these attitudes could seriously limit their ability to slow the spread of infection in the population. AIDS is an unusual problem, they say, and it requires unusual and innovative solutions.

The history of sex education in this country suggests that the question of who should develop and pay for education to reduce risk will remain controversial. A significant portion of this responsibility probably will be assumed by the private sector. The only certainty is that education and other public health measures are now the only methods available to control transmission of AIDS.

Conclusion

AIDS is the most complex public health challenge confronting modern medicine. The characteristics of the virus place it just out of reach of the most advanced therapeutic drugs. At a time when policymakers at every level have called for a reduction in health care spending, AIDS imposes a massive financial burden. In a period characterized by tolerance of unconventional life-styles, AIDS provokes calls for quarantine and other restrictive measures.

Questions of public responsibility arising from the syndrome are endless. Examples include:

• How should funds be divided among competing research needs?
• Who should bear the costs of patient care?
• Should insurance companies be permitted to screen for HTLV-III/LAV antibodies?
• How should the courts handle liability for transfusion-associated AIDS?
• What are the rights of AIDS victims in the workplace?
• How should employers deal with co-workers who refuse to work with AIDS patients?
• Is mandatory testing a necessity or an invasion of privacy?

The breadth of these questions underscores the fact that AIDS affects everybody, not just those who adhere to a particular life-style or who live in a certain part of the country. Government officials at all levels, business leaders, educators, health care professionals, and everyone else who cares about how our society balances the needs of the community against those of individuals should participate in the development of reasonable and equitable approaches to the AIDS crisis.

*   *   *

Chapter 8 is based on the presentations of Mervyn F. Silverman, consultant and former Director of Health for San Francisco; Brett J. Cassens, American Association of Physicians for Human Rights; Philip R. Lee, Institute for Health Policy Studies, University of California at San Francisco; Ronald Bayer, The Hastings Center; and June E. Osborn, School of Public Health, University of Michigan.

Appendixes

Suggested Readings

Glossary

Contributors and Acknowledgments

Index

Appendix A

Current CDC Definition of AIDS

For the limited purposes of national reporting of some of the severe late manifestations of infection with human T-lymphotropic virus, type-III/lymphadenopathy-associated virus (HTLV-III/LAV) in the United States, CDC defines a case of "acquired immunodeficiency syndrome" (AIDS) as an illness characterized by:

I. one or more of the opportunistic diseases listed below (diagnosed by methods considered reliable) that are at least moderately indicative of underlying cellular immunodeficiency, and

II. absence of all known underlying causes of cellular immunodeficiency (other than HTLV-III/LAV infection) and absence of all other causes of reduced resistance reported to be associated with at least one of those opportunistic diseases.

Despite having the above, patients are excluded as AIDS cases if they have negative result(s) on testing for serum antibody to HTLV-III/LAV,* do not have a positive culture for HTLV-III/LAV,

---

Source: Reprinted from "The Case Definition of AIDS Used by CDC for National Reporting (CDC-reportable AIDS)," Document No. 0312S, August 1, 1985, Centers for Disease Control, Atlanta, Ga.

*A single negative test for HTLV-III/LAV may be applied here if it is an antibody test by ELISA, immunofluorescent, or Western Blot methods, because such tests are very sensitive. Viral cultures are less sensitive but more specific, and so may be relied on if positive but not if negative. If multiple antibody tests have inconsistent results, the result applied to the case definition should be that of the majority. A positive culture, however, would over-rule negative antibody tests.

and have both a normal or high number of T-helper (OKT4 or LEU3) lymphocytes and a normal or high ratio of T-helper to T-suppressor (OKT8 or LEU2) lymphocytes. In the absence of test results, patients satisfying all other criteria in this definition are included as cases.

This general case definition may be made more explicit by specifying:

I.   the particular diseases considered at least moderately indicative of cellular immunodeficiency, which are used as indicators of AIDS, and

II. the known causes of cellular immunodeficiency, or other causes of reduced resistance reported to be associated with particular diseases, which would disqualify a patient as an AIDS case.

This specification is as follows:

I. **Diseases at least moderately indicative of underlying cellular immunodeficiency:**

In the following list of diseases, the required diagnostic methods with positive results are shown in parentheses. "Microscopy" may include cytology.

A. *Protozoal and Helminthic Infections:*
1. Cryptosporidiosis, intestinal, causing diarrhea for over 1 month (on histology or stool microscopy)
2. *Pneumocystis carinii* pneumonia (on histology, or microscopy of a "touch" preparation, bronchial washings, or sputum)
3. Strongyloidosis, causing pneumonia, central nervous system infection, or infection disseminated beyond the gastrointestinal tract (on histology)
4. Toxoplasmosis, causing infection in internal organs other than liver, spleen, or lymph nodes (on histology or microscopy of a "touch" preparation)

B. *Fungal Infections:*
1. Candidiasis, causing esophagitis (on histology, or microscopy of a "wet" preparation from the esophagus, or endoscopic or autopsy findings of white plaques on an erythematous mucosal base, but not by culture alone)

2. Cryptococcosis, causing central nervous system or other infection disseminated beyond lungs and lymph nodes (on culture, antigen detection, histology, or India ink preparation of CSF)

C. *Bacterial Infections:*
1. *Mycobacterium avium* or *intracellulare* (*Mycobacterium avium* complex), or *Mycobacterium kansasii*, causing infection disseminated beyond lungs and lymph nodes (on culture)

D. *Viral Infections:*
1. Cytomegalovirus, causing infection in internal organs other than liver, spleen, or lymph nodes (on histology or cytology, but not by culture or serum antibody titer)
2. Herpes simplex virus, causing chronic mucocutaneous infection with ulcers persisting more than 1 month, or pulmonary, gastrointestinal tract (beyond mouth, throat, or rectum), or disseminated infection (but not encephalitis alone) (on culture, histology, or cytology)
3. Progressive multifocal leukoencephalopathy (presumed to be caused by Papovavirus) (on histology)

E. *Cancer:*
1. Kaposi's sarcoma (on histology)
2. Lymphoma limited to the brain (on histology)

F. *Other Opportunistic Infections with Positive Test for HTLV-III/LAV*:*

In the absence of the above opportunistic diseases, any of the following diseases is considered indicative of AIDS if the patient had a positive test for HTLV-III/LAV*:

1. disseminated histoplasmosis (on culture, histology, or cytology)
2. bronchial or pulmonary candidiasis (on microscopy or

---

*A positive test for HTLV-III/LAV may consist of a reactive test for antibody to HTLV-III/LAV or a positive culture (isolation of HTLV-III/LAV from a culture of the patient's peripheral blood lymphocytes). If multiple antibody tests have inconsistent results, the result applied to the case definition should be that of the majority done by the ELISA, immunofluorescent, or Western Blot methods. A positive culture, however, would over-rule negative antibody tests.

visualization grossly of characteristic white plaques on the bronchial mucosa, but not by culture alone)
3. isosporiasis, causing chronic diarrhea (over 1 month), (on histology or stool microscopy)

G. *Chronic lymphoid interstitial pneumonitis:*
In the absence of the above opportunistic diseases, a histologically confirmed diagnosis of chronic (persisting over 2 months) lymphoid interstitial pneumonitis in a child (under 13 years of age) is indicative of AIDS unless test(s) for HTLV-III/LAV are negative.* The histologic examination of lung tissue must show diffuse interstitial and peribronchiolar infiltration by lymphocytes, plasma cells with Russell bodies, plasmacytoid lymphocytes and immunoblasts. Histologic and culture evaluation must not identify a pathogenic organism as the cause of this pneumonia.

H. *Non-Hodgkin's Lymphoma with Positive Test for HTLV-III/LAV*:*
If the patient had a positive test for HTLV-III/LAV,* then the following histologic types of lymphoma are indicative of AIDS, regardless of anatomic site:

1. Small *non*cleaved lymphoma (Burkitt's tumor or Burkitt-like lymphoma), but not small cleaved lymphoma,
2. Immunoblastic sarcoma (or immunoblastic lymphoma) of B-cell or unknown immunologic phenotype (not of T-cell type). Other terms which may be equivalent include: diffuse undifferentiated non-Hodgkin's lymphoma, large cell lymphoma (cleaved or noncleaved), diffuse histiocytic lymphoma, reticulum cell sarcoma, and high-grade lymphoma.

Lymphomas should not be accepted as indicative of AIDS if they are described in any of the following ways: low grade, of T-cell type (immunologic phenotype), small cleaved lymphoma, lymphocytic lymphoma (regardless of whether well or poorly differentiated), lymphoblastic lymphoma, plasmacytoid lymphocytic lymphoma, lymphocytic leukemia (acute or chronic), or Hodgkin's disease (or Hodgkin's lymphoma).

---

*See footnote on p. 151.

II.   Known Causes of Reduced Resistance:

Known causes of reduced resistance to diseases indicative of immunodeficiency are listed in the left column, while the diseases that may be attributable to these causes (rather than to the immunodeficiency caused by HTLV-III/LAV infection) are listed on the right:

Known Causes of Reduced Resistance

Diseases Possibly Attributable to the Known Causes of Reduced Resistance

1. Systemic corticosteroid therapy

Any infection diagnosed during or within 1 month after discontinuation of the corticosteroid therapy, unless symptoms specific for an infected anatomic site (e.g., dyspnea for pneumonia, headache for encephalitis, diarrhea for colitis) began before the corticosteroid therapy

or any cancer diagnosed during or within 1 month after discontinuation of more than 4 months of long-term corticosteroid therapy, unless symptoms specific for the anatomic sites of the cancer (as described above) began before the long-term corticosteroid therapy

2. Other immunosuppressive or cytotoxic therapy

Any infection diagnosed during or within 1 year after discontinuation of the immunosuppressive therapy, unless symptoms specific for an infected anatomic site (as described above) began before the therapy or any cancer diagnosed during or within 1 year after discontinuation of more than 4 months of long-term immunosuppressive therapy, unless symptoms specific for the anatomic sites of the cancer (as described above) began before the long-term therapy

3. Cancer of lymphoreticular or histiocytic tissue such as lymphoma (except for lymphoma localized to the brain), Hodgkin's disease, lymphocytic leukemia, or multiple myeloma

Any infection or cancer, if diagnosed after or within 3 months before the diagnosis of the cancer of lymphoreticular or histiocytic tissue

4. Age 60 years or older at diagnosis

Kaposi's sarcoma, but not if the patient has a positive test for HTLV-III/LAV

5. Age under 28 days (neonatal) at diagnosis

Toxoplasmosis or herpes simplex virus infection, as described above

6. Age under 6 months at diagnosis

Cytomegalovirus infection, as described above

7. An immunodeficiency atypical of AIDS, such as one involving hypogammaglobulinemia or angioimmunoblastic lymphadenopathy; or an immunodeficiency of which the cause appears to be a genetic or developmental defect, rather than HTLV-III/LAV infection

Any infection or cancer diagnosed during such immunodeficiency

8. Exogenous malnutrition (starvation due to food deprivation, not malnutrition due to malabsorption or illness)

Any infection or cancer diagnosed during or within 1 month after discontinuation of starvation

Appendix B

PHS Recommendations for Preventing Transmission of Infection with HTLV–III/LAV in the Workplace

Summary

The information and recommendations contained in this document have been developed with particular emphasis on health-care workers and others in related occupations in which exposure might occur to blood from persons infected with HTLV–III/LAV, the "AIDS virus." Because of public concern about the purported risk of transmission of HTLV–III/LAV by persons providing personal services and those preparing and serving food and beverages, this document also addresses personal-service and food-service workers. Finally, it addresses "other workers"—persons in settings, such as offices, schools, factories, and construction sites, where there is no known risk of AIDS virus transmission.

Because AIDS is a bloodborne, sexually transmitted disease that is not spread by casual contact, this document does *not* recommend routine HTLV–III/LAV antibody screening for the groups addressed. Because AIDS is not transmitted through preparation or serving of food and beverages, these recommendations state that food-service workers known to be infected with AIDS should not be restricted from work unless they have another infection or illness for which such restriction would be warranted.

This document contains detailed recommendations for precautions appropriate to prevent transmission of all blood-borne infectious diseases to people exposed—in the course of

Source: Reprinted from *Morbidity and Mortality Weekly Report*, Vol. 34, No. 45 (Nov. 15, 1985), pp. 681–695.

their duties—to blood from persons who may be infected with HTLV-III/LAV. They emphasize that health-care workers should take all possible precautions to prevent needlestick injury. The recommendations are based on the well-documented modes of HTLV-III/LAV transmission and incorporate a "worst case" scenario, the hepatitis B model of transmission. Because the hepatitis B virus is also bloodborne and is both hardier and more infectious than HTLV-III/LAV, recommendations that would prevent transmission of hepatitis B will also prevent transmission of AIDS.

Formulation of specific recommendations for health-care workers who perform invasive procedures is in progress.

Persons at increased risk of acquiring infection with human T-lymphotropic virus type III/lymphadenopathy-associated virus (HTLV-III/LAV), the virus that causes acquired immunodeficiency syndrome (AIDS), include homosexual and bisexual men, intravenous (IV) drug abusers, persons transfused with contaminated blood or blood products, heterosexual contacts of persons with HTLV-III/LAV infection, and children born to infected mothers. HTLV-III/LAV is transmitted through sexual contact, parenteral exposure to infected blood or blood components, and perinatal transmission from mother to neonate. HTLV-III/LAV has been isolated from blood, semen, saliva, tears, breast milk, and urine and is likely to be isolated from some other body fluids, secretions, and excretions, but epidemiologic evidence has implicated only blood and semen in transmission. Studies of nonsexual household contacts of AIDS patients indicate that casual contact with saliva and tears does not result in transmission of infection. Spread of infection to household contacts of infected persons has not been detected when the household contacts have not been sex partners or have not been infants of infected mothers. The kind of nonsexual person-to-person contact that generally occurs among workers and clients or consumers in the workplace does not pose a risk for transmission of HTLV-III/LAV.

As in the development of any such recommendations, the paramount consideration is the protection of the public's health. The following recommendations have been developed for all workers, particularly workers in occupations in which exposure might occur to blood from individuals infected with HTLV-III/LAV. These recommendations reinforce and supplement the specific recommendations that were published earlier for clinical and laboratory staffs (1) and for dental-care personnel and persons performing necropsies and morticians' services (2). Because of public concern about the

purported risk of transmission of HTLV-III/LAV by persons providing personal services and by food and beverages, these recommendations contain information and recommendations for personal-
service and food-service workers. Finally, these recommendations
address workplaces in general where there is no known risk of
transmission of HTLV-III/LAV (e.g., offices, schools, factories,
construction sites). Formulation of specific recommendations for
health-care workers (HCWs) who perform invasive procedures
(e.g., surgeons, dentists) is in progress. Separate recommendations
are also being developed to prevent HTLV-III/LAV transmission in
prisons, other correctional facilities, and institutions housing individuals who may exhibit uncontrollable behavior (e.g., custodial
institutions) and in the perinatal setting. In addition, separate recommendations have already been developed for children in schools
and day-care centers (3).

HTLV-III/LAV-infected individuals include those with AIDS
(4); those diagnosed by their physician(s) as having other illnesses
due to infection with HTLV-III/LAV; and those who have virologic
or serologic evidence of infection with HTLV-III/LAV but who are
not ill.

These recommendations are based on the well-documented
modes of HTLV-III/LAV transmission identified in epidemiologic
studies and on comparison with the hepatitis B experience. Other
recommendations are based on the hepatitis B model of transmission.

Comparison with the Hepatitis B Virus Experience

The epidemiology of HTLV-III/LAV infection is similar to that
of hepatitis B virus (HBV) infection, and much that has been learned
over the last 15 years related to the risk of acquiring hepatitis B in the
workplace can be applied to understanding the risk of HTLV-
III/LAV transmission in the health-care and other occupational
settings. Both viruses are transmitted through sexual contact, parenteral exposure to contaminated blood or blood products, and
perinatal transmission from infected mothers to their offspring.
Thus, some of the same major groups at high risk for HBV infection
(e.g., homosexual men, IV drug abusers, persons with hemophilia,
infants born to infected mothers) are also the groups at highest risk
for HTLV-III/LAV infection. Neither HBV nor HTLV-III/LAV has
been shown to be transmitted by casual contact in the workplace,
contaminated food or water, or airborne or fecal-oral routes (5).

HBV infection is an occupational risk for HCWs, but this risk is related to degree of contact with blood or contaminated needles. HCWs who do not have contact with blood or needles contaminated with blood are not at risk for acquiring HBV infection in the workplace (6–8).

In the health-care setting, HBV transmission has not been documented between hospitalized patients, except in hemodialysis units, where blood contamination of the environment has been extensive or where HBV-positive blood from one patient has been transferred to another patient through contamination of instruments. Evidence of HBV transmission from HCWs to patients has been rare and limited to situations in which the HCWs exhibited high concentrations of virus in their blood (at least 100,000,000 infectious virus particles per ml of serum), and the HCWs sustained a puncture wound while performing traumatic procedures on patients or had exudative or weeping lesions that allowed virus to contaminate instruments or open wounds of patients (9–11).

Current evidence indicates that, despite epidemiologic similarities of HBV and HTLV-III/LAV infection, the risk for HBV transmission in health-care settings far exceeds that for HTLV-III/LAV transmission. The risk of acquiring HBV infection following a needlestick from an HBV carrier ranges from 6% to 30% (12,13), far in excess of the risk of HTLV-III/LAV infection following a needlestick involving a source patient infected with HTLV-III/LAV, which is less than 1%. In addition, all HCWs who have been shown to transmit HBV infection in health-care settings have belonged to the subset of chronic HBV carriers who, when tested, have exhibited evidence of exceptionally high concentrations of virus (at least 100,000,000 infectious virus particles per ml) in their blood. Chronic carriers who have substantially lower concentrations of virus in their blood have not been implicated in transmission in the health-care setting (9–11,14). The HBV model thus represents a "worst case" condition in regard to transmission in health-care and other related settings. Therefore, recommendations for the control of HBV infection should, if followed, also effectively prevent spread of HTLV-III/LAV. Whether additional measures are indicated for those HCWs who perform invasive procedures will be addressed in the recommendations currently being developed.

Routine screening of all patients or HCWs for evidence of HBV infection has never been recommended. Control of HBV transmission in the health-care setting has emphasized the implementation of recommendations for the appropriate handling of blood, other body fluids, and items soiled with blood or other body fluids.

Transmission from Patients to Health-Care Workers

HCWs include, but are not limited to, nurses, physicians, dentists and other dental workers, optometrists, podiatrists, chiropractors, laboratory and blood bank technologists and technicians, phlebotomists, dialysis personnel, paramedics, emergency medical technicians, medical examiners, morticians, housekeepers, laundry workers, and others whose work involves contact with patients, their blood or other body fluids, or corpses.

Recommendations for HCWs emphasize precautions appropriate for preventing transmission of bloodborne infectious diseases, including HTLV-III/LAV and HBV infections. Thus, these precautions should be enforced routinely, as should other standard infection-control precautions, regardless of whether HCWs or patients are known to be infected with HTLV-III/LAV or HBV. In addition to being informed of these precautions, all HCWs, including students and housestaff, should be educated regarding the epidemiology, modes of transmission, and prevention of HTLV-III/LAV infection.

Risk of HCWs Acquiring HTLV-III/LAV in the Workplace   Using the HBV model, the highest risk for transmission of HTLV-III/LAV in the workplace would involve parenteral exposure to a needle or other sharp instrument contaminated with blood of an infected patient. The risk to HCWs of acquiring HTLV-III/LAV infection in the workplace has been evaluated in several studies. In five separate studies, a total of 1,498 HCWs have been tested for antibody to HTLV-III/LAV. In these studies, 666 (44.5%) of the HCWs had direct parenteral (needlestick or cut) or mucous membrane exposure to patients with AIDS or HTLV-III/LAV infection. Most of these exposures were to blood rather than to other body fluids. None of the HCWs whose initial serologic tests were negative developed subsequent evidence of HTLV-III/LAV infection following their exposures. Twenty-six HCWs in these five studies were seropositive when first tested; all but three of these persons belonged to groups recognized to be at increased risk for AIDS (15). Since one was tested anonymously, epidemiologic information was available on only two of these three seropositive HCWs. Although these two

HCWs were reported as probable occupationally related HTLV-III/LAV infection (*15,16*), neither had a preexposure nor an early postexposure serum sample available to help determine the onset of infection. One case reported from England describes a nurse who seroconverted following an accidental parenteral exposure to a needle contaminated with blood from an AIDS patient (*17*).

In spite of the extremely low risk of transmission of HTLV-III/LAV infection, even when needlestick injuries occur, more emphasis must be given to precautions targeted to prevent needlestick injuries in HCWs caring for any patient, since such injuries continue to occur even during the care of patients who are known to be infected with HTLV-III/LAV.

Precautions to Prevent Acquisition of HTLV-III/LAV Infection by HCWs in the Workplace   These precautions represent prudent practices that apply to preventing transmission of HTLV-III/LAV and other bloodborne infections and should be used routinely (*18*).

1. Sharp items (needles, scalpel blades, and other sharp instruments) should be considered as potentially infective and be handled with extraordinary care to prevent accidental injuries.

2. Disposable syringes and needles, scalpel blades, and other sharp items should be placed into puncture-resistant containers located as close as practical to the area in which they were used. To prevent needlestick injuries, needles should not be recapped, purposefully bent, broken, removed from disposable syringes, or otherwise manipulated by hand.

3. When the possibility of exposure to blood or other body fluids exists, routinely recommended precautions should be followed. The anticipated exposure may require gloves alone, as in handling items soiled with blood or equipment contaminated with blood or other body fluids, or may also require gowns, masks, and eye-coverings when performing procedures involving more extensive contact with blood or potentially infective body fluids, as in some dental or endoscopic procedures or postmortem examinations. Hands should be washed thoroughly and immediately if they accidentally become contaminated with blood.

4. To minimize the need for emergency mouth-to-mouth resuscitation, mouth pieces, resuscitation bags, or other ventilation devices should be strategically located and available for use in areas where the need for resuscitation is predictable.

5. Pregnant HCWs are not known to be at greater risk of

contracting HTLV-III/LAV infections than HCWs who are not pregnant; however, if a HCW develops HTLV-III/LAV infection during pregnancy, the infant is at increased risk of infection resulting from perinatal transmission. Because of this risk, pregnant HCWs should be especially familiar with precautions for preventing HTLV-III/LAV transmission (*19*).

Precautions for HCWs During Home Care of Persons Infected with HTLV-III/LAV Persons infected with HTLV-III/LAV can be safely cared for in home environments. Studies of family members of patients infected with HTLV-III/LAV have found no evidence of HTLV-III/LAV transmission to adults who were not sexual contacts of the infected patients or to children who were not at risk for perinatal transmission (*3*). HCWs providing home care face the same risk of transmission of infection as HCWs in hospitals and other health-care settings, especially if there are needlesticks or other parenteral or mucous membrane exposures to blood or other body fluids.

When providing health-care service in the home to persons infected with HTLV-III/LAV, measures similar to those used in hospitals are appropriate. As in the hospital, needles should not be recapped, purposefully bent, broken, removed from disposable syringes, or otherwise manipulated by hand. Needles and other sharp items should be placed into puncture-resistant containers and disposed of in accordance with local regulations for solid waste. Blood and other body fluids can be flushed down the toilet. Other items for disposal that are contaminated with blood or other body fluids that cannot be flushed down the toilet should be wrapped securely in a plastic bag that is impervious and sturdy (not easily penetrated). It should be placed in a second bag before being discarded in a manner consistent with local regulations for solid waste disposal. Spills of blood or other body fluids should be cleaned with soap and water or a household detergent. As in the hospital, individuals cleaning up such spills should wear disposable gloves. A disinfectant solution or a freshly prepared solution of sodium hypochlorite (household bleach, see below) should be used to wipe the area after cleaning.

Precautions for Providers of Prehospital Emergency Health Care Providers of prehospital emergency health care include the following: paramedics, emergency medical technicians, law enforcement personnel, firefighters, lifeguards, and others whose job might require them to provide first-response medical care. The risk of transmission of infection, including HTLV-III/LAV infection, from infected persons to providers of prehospital emergency health care should be no higher than that for HCWs providing emergency care in the hospital if appropriate precautions are taken to prevent exposure to blood or other body fluids.

Providers of prehospital emergency health care should follow the precautions outlined above for other HCWs. No transmission of HBV infection during mouth-to-mouth resuscitation has been documented. However, because of the theoretical risk of salivary transmission of HTLV-III/LAV during mouth-to-mouth resuscitation, special attention should be given to the use of disposable airway equipment or resuscitation bags and the wearing of gloves when in contact with blood or other body fluids. Resuscitation equipment and devices known or suspected to be contaminated with blood or other body fluids should be used once and disposed of or be thoroughly cleaned and disinfected after each use.

Management of Parenteral and Mucous Membrane Exposures of HCWs   If a HCW has a parenteral (e.g., needlestick or cut) or mucous membrane (e.g., splash to the eye or mouth) exposure to blood or other body fluids, the source patient should be assessed clinically and epidemiologically to determine the likelihood of HTLV-III/LAV infection. If the assessment suggests that infection may exist, the patient should be informed of the incident and requested to consent to serologic testing for evidence of HTLV-III/LAV infection. If the source patient has AIDS or other evidence of HTLV-III/LAV infection, declines testing, or has a positive test, the HCW should be evaluated clinically and serologically for evidence of HTLV-III/LAV infection as soon as possible after the exposure, and, if seronegative, retested after 6 weeks and on a periodic basis thereafter (e.g., 3, 6, and 12 months following exposure) to determine if transmission has occurred. During this follow-up period, especially the first 6–12 weeks, when most infected persons are expected to seroconvert, exposed HCWs should receive counseling about the risk of infection and follow U.S. Public Health Service (PHS) recommendations for preventing transmission of AIDS (20,21). If the source patient is seronegative and has no other evidence of HTLV-III/LAV infection, no further follow-up of the HCW is necessary. If the source patient cannot be identified, decisions regarding appropriate follow-up should be individualized based on the type of exposure and the likelihood that the source patient was infected.

Serologic Testing of Patients   Routine serologic testing of all patients for antibody to HTLV-III/LAV is not recommended to prevent transmission of HTLV-III/LAV infection in the workplace. Results of such testing are unlikely to further reduce the risk of transmission, which, even with documented needlesticks, is already extremely low. Furthermore, the risk of needlestick and other parenteral exposures could be reduced by emphasizing and more consistently implementing routinely recommended infection-control precautions (e.g., not recapping needles). Moreover, results of routine serologic testing would not be available for emergency cases and patients with short lengths of stay, and additional tests to determine whether a positive test was a true or false positive would be required in populations with a low prevalence of infection. However, this recommendation is based only on considerations of occupational risks and should not be construed as a recommendation against other uses of the serologic test, such as for diagnosis or to facilitate medical management of patients. Since the experience with infected patients varies substantially among hospitals (75% of all AIDS cases have been reported by only 280 of the more than 6,000 acute-care hospitals in the United States), some hospitals in certain geographic areas may deem it appropriate to initiate serologic testing of patients.

Transmission from Health-Care Workers to Patients

Risk of Transmission of HTLV-III/LAV Infection from HCWs to Patients   Although there is no evidence that HCWs infected with HTLV-III/LAV have transmitted infection to patients, a risk of transmission of HTLV-III/LAV infection from HCWs to patients would exist in situations where there is both (1) a high degree of trauma to the patient that would provide a portal of entry for the virus (e.g., during invasive procedures) and (2) access of blood or serous fluid from the infected HCW to the open tissue of a patient, as could occur if the HCW sustains a needlestick or scalpel injury during an invasive procedure. HCWs known to be infected with

HTLV-III/LAV who do not perform invasive procedures need not be restricted from work unless they have evidence of other infection or illness for which any HCW should be restricted. Whether additional restrictions are indicated for HCWs who perform invasive procedures is currently being considered.

Precautions to Prevent Transmission of HTLV-III/LAV Infection from HCWs to Patients These precautions apply to all HCWs, regardless of whether they perform invasive procedures: (1) All HCWs should wear gloves for direct contact with mucous membranes or nonintact skin of all patients and (2) HCWs who have exudative lesions or weeping dermatitis should refrain from all direct patient care and from handling patient-care equipment until the condition resolves.

Management of Parenteral and Mucous Membrane Exposures of Patients If a patient has a parenteral or mucous membrane exposure to blood or other body fluids of a HCW, the patient should be informed of the incident and the same procedure outlined above for exposures of HCWs to patients should be followed for both the source HCW and the potentially exposed patient. Management of this type of exposure will be addressed in more detail in the recommendations for HCWs who perform invasive procedures.

Serologic Testing of HCWs Routine serologic testing of HCWs who do not perform invasive procedures (including providers of home and prehospital emergency care) is not recommended to prevent transmission of HTLV-III/LAV infection. The risk of transmission is extremely low and can be further minimized when routinely recommended infection–control precautions are followed. However, serologic testing should be available to HCWs who may wish to know their HTLV-III/LAV infection status. Whether indications exist for serologic testing of HCWs who perform invasive procedures is currently being considered.

Risk of Occupational Acquisition of Other Infectious Diseases by HCWs Infected with HTLV-III/LAV HCWs who are known to be infected with HTLV-III/LAV and who have defective immune systems are at increased risk of acquiring or experiencing serious complications of other infectious diseases. Of particular concern is the risk of severe infection following exposure to patients with infectious diseases that are easily transmitted if appropriate precautions are not taken (e.g., tuberculosis). HCWs infected with HTLV-III/LAV should be counseled about the potential risk associated with taking care of patients with transmissible infections and should continue to follow existing recommendations for infection control to minimize their risk of exposure to other infectious agents (*18,19*). The HCWs' personal physician(s), in conjunction with their institutions' personnel health services or medical directors, should determine on an individual basis whether the infected HCWs can adequately and safely perform patient-care duties and suggest changes in work assignments, if indicated. In making this determination, recommendations of the Immunization Practices Advisory Committee and institutional policies concerning requirements for vaccinating HCWs with live-virus vaccines should also be considered.

Sterilization, Disinfection, Housekeeping, and Waste Disposal to Prevent Transmission of HTLV-III/LAV

Sterilization and disinfection procedures currently recommended for use (*22,23*) in health-care and dental facilities are adequate to sterilize or disinfect instruments, devices, or other items contaminated with the blood or other body fluids from individuals infected with HTLV-III/LAV. Instruments or other nondisposable items that enter normally sterile tissue or the vascular system or through which blood flows should be sterilized before reuse. Surgical instruments used on all patients should be decontaminated after use rather than just rinsed with water. Decontamination can be accomplished by machine or by hand cleaning by trained personnel wearing appropriate protective attire (*24*) and using appropriate chemical germicides. Instruments or other nondisposable items that touch intact mucous membranes should receive high-level disinfection.

Several liquid chemical germicides commonly used in laboratories and health-care facilities have been shown to kill HTLV-III/LAV at concentrations much lower than are used in practice (*25*). When decontaminating instruments or medical devices, chemical germicides that are registered with and approved by the U.S. Environmental Protection Agency (EPA) as "sterilants" can be used either for sterilization or for high-level disinfection depending on contact time; germicides that are approved for use as "hospital disinfectants" and are mycobactericidal when used at appropriate dilutions can also be used for high-level disinfection of devices and instruments. Germicides that are mycobactericidal are preferred because mycobacteria represent one of the most resistant groups of microorganisms; therefore, germicides that are effective against mycobacteria are also effective against other bacterial and viral pathogens. When chemical germicides are used, instruments or devices to be sterilized or disinfected should be thoroughly cleaned before exposure to the germicide, and the manufacturer's instructions for use of the germicide should be followed.

Laundry and dishwashing cycles commonly used in hospitals are adequate to decontaminate linens, dishes, glassware, and utensils. When cleaning environmental surfaces, housekeeping procedures commonly used in hospitals are adequate; surfaces exposed to blood and body fluids should be cleaned with a detergent followed by decontamination using an EPA-approved hospital disinfectant that is mycobactericidal. Individuals cleaning up such spills should wear disposable gloves. Information on specific label claims of commercial germicides can be obtained by writing to the Disinfectants Branch, Office of Pesticides, Environmental Protection Agency, 401 M Street, S.W., Washington, D.C., 20460.

In addition to hospital disinfectants, a freshly prepared solution of sodium hypochlorite (household bleach) is an inexpensive and very effective germicide (25). Concentrations ranging from 5,000 ppm (a 1:10 dilution of household bleach) to 500 ppm (a 1:100 dilution) sodium hypochlorite are effective, depending on the amount of organic material (e.g., blood, mucus, etc.) present on the surface to be cleaned and disinfected.

Sharp items should be considered as potentially infective and should be handled and disposed of with extraordinary care to prevent accidental injuries. Other potentially infective waste should be contained and transported in clearly identified impervious plastic bags. If the outside of the bag is contaminated with blood or other body fluids, a second outer bag should be used. Recommended practices for disposal of infective waste (23) are adequate for disposal of waste contaminated by HTLV-III/LAV. Blood and other body fluids may be carefully poured down a drain connected to a sanitary sewer.

Considerations Relevant to Other Workers

Personal-Service Workers (PSWs)   PSWs are defined as individuals whose occupations involve close personal contact with clients (e.g., hairdressers, barbers, estheticians, cosmetologists, manicurists, pedicurists, massage therapists). PSWs whose services (tattooing, ear piercing, acupuncture, etc.) require needles or other instruments that penetrate the skin should follow precautions indicated for HCWs. Although there is no evidence of transmission of HTLV-III/LAV from clients to PSWs, from PSWs to clients, or between clients of PSWs, a risk of transmission would exist from PSWs to clients and vice versa in situations where there is both (1) trauma to one of the individuals that would provide a portal of entry for the virus and (2) access of blood or serous fluid from one infected person to the open tissue of the other, as could occur if either sustained a cut. A risk of transmission from client to client exists when instruments contaminated with blood are not sterilized or disinfected between clients. However, HBV transmission has been documented only rarely in acupuncture, ear piercing, and tattoo establishments and never in other personal-service settings, indicating that any risk for HTLV-III/LAV transmission in personal-service settings must be extremely low.

All PSWs should be educated about transmission of bloodborne infections, including HTLV-III/LAV and HBV. Such education should emphasize principles of good hygiene, antisepsis, and disinfection. This education can be accomplished by national or state professional organizations, with assistance from state and local health departments, using lectures at meetings or self-instructional materials. Licensure requirements should include evidence of such education. Instruments that are intended to penetrate the skin (e.g., tattooing and acupuncture needles, ear piercing devices) should be used once and disposed of or be thoroughly cleaned and sterilized after each use using procedures recommended for use in health-care institutions. Instruments not intended to penetrate the skin but which may become contaminated with blood (e.g., razors), should be used for only one client and be disposed of or thoroughly cleaned and disinfected after use using procedures recommended for use in health-care institutions. Any PSW with exudative lesions or weeping dermatitis, regardless of HTLV-III/LAV infection status, should refrain from direct contact with clients until the condition resolves. PSWs known to be infected with HTLV-III/LAV need not be restricted from work unless they have evidence of other infections or illnesses for which any PSW should also be restricted.

Routine serologic testing of PSWs for antibody to HTLV-III/LAV is not recommended to prevent transmission from PSWs to clients.

Food-Service Workers (FSWs)   FSWs are defined as individuals whose occupations involve the preparation or serving of food or beverages (e.g., cooks, caterers, servers, waiters, bartenders, airline attendants). All epidemiologic and laboratory evidence indicates that bloodborne and sexually transmitted infections are not transmitted during the preparation or serving of food or beverages, and no instances of HBV or HTLV-III/LAV transmission have been documented in this setting.

All FSWs should follow recommended standards and practices of good personal hygiene and food sanitation (*26*). All FSWs should exercise care to avoid injury to hands when preparing food. Should such an injury occur, both aesthetic and sanitary conditions would dictate that food contaminated with blood be discarded. FSWs known to be infected with HTLV-III/LAV need not be restricted from work unless they have evidence of other infection or illness for which any FSW should also be restricted.

Routine serologic testing of FSWs for antibody to HTLV-III/LAV is not recommended to prevent disease transmission from FSWs to consumers.

Other Workers Sharing the Same Work Environment   No known risk of transmission to co-workers, clients, or consumers exists from HTLV-III/LAV-infected workers in other settings (e.g., offices, schools, factories, construction sites). This infection is spread by sexual contact with infected persons, injection of contaminated blood or blood products, and by perinatal transmission. Workers known to be infected with HTLV-III/LAV should not be restricted from work solely based on this finding. Moreover, they should not be restricted from using telephones, office equipment, toilets, showers, eating facilities, and water fountains. Equipment contaminated with blood or other body fluids of any workers, regardless of HTLV-III/LAV infection status, should be cleaned with soap and water or a detergent. A disinfectant solution or a fresh solution of sodium hypochlorite (household bleach, see above) should be used to wipe the area after cleaning.

Other Issues in the Workplace

The information and recommendations contained in this document do not address all the potential issues that may have to be considered when making specific employment decisions for persons with HTLV-III/LAV infection. The diagnosis of HTLV-III/LAV infection may evoke unwarranted fear and suspicion in some co-workers. Other issues that may be considered include the need for confidentiality, applicable federal, state, or local laws governing occupational safety and health, civil rights of employees, workers' compensation laws, provisions of collective bargaining agreements, confidentiality of medical records, informed consent, employee and patient privacy rights, and employee right-to-know statutes.

Development of These Recommendations

The information and recommendations contained in these recommendations were developed and compiled by CDC and other PHS agencies in consultation with individuals representing various organizations. The following organizations were represented: Association of State and Territorial Health Officials, Conference of State and Territorial Epidemiologists, Association of State and Territorial Public Health Laboratory Directors, National Association of County Health Officials, American Hospital Association, United States Conference of Local Health Officers, Association for Practitioners in Infection Control, Society of Hospital Epidemiologists of America, American Dental Association, American Medical Association, American Nurses' Association, American Association of Medical Colleges, American Association of Dental Schools, National Institutes of Health, Food and Drug Administration, Food Research Institute, National Restaurant Association, National Hairdressers and Cosmetologists Association, National Gay Task Force, National Funeral Directors and Morticians Association, American Association of Physicians for Human Rights, and National Association of Emergency Medical Technicians. The consultants also included a labor union representative, an attorney, a corporate medical director, and a pathologist. However, these recommendations may not reflect the views of individual consultants or the organizations they represented.

References

1. CDC. Acquired immune deficiency syndrome (AIDS): precautions for clinical and laboratory staffs. MMWR 1982;31:577–80.
2. CDC. Acquired immunodeficiency syndrome (AIDS): precautions for health-care workers and allied professionals. MMWR 1983;32:450–1.

3. CDC. Education and foster care of children infected with human T-lymphotropic virus type III/lymphadenopathy-associated virus. MMWR 1985;34:517–21.

4. CDC. Revision of the case definition of acquired immunodeficiency syndrome for national reporting—United States. MMWR 1985;34:373–5.

5. CDC. ACIP recommendations for protection against viral hepatitis. MMWR 1985;34:313–24, 329–335.

6. Hadler SC, Doto IL, Maynard JE, et al. Occupational risk of hepatitis B infection in hospital workers. Infect Control 1985;6:24–31.

7. Dienstag JL, Ryan DM. Occupational exposure to hepatitis B virus in hospital personnel: infection or immunization? Am J Epidemiol 1982;115:26–39.

8. Pattison CP, Maynard JE, Berquist KR, et al. Epidemiology of hepatitis B in hospital personnel. Am J Epidemiol 1975;101:59–64.

9. Kane MA, Lettau LA. Transmission of HBV from dental personnel to patients. JADA 1985;110:634–6.

10. Hadler SC, Sorley DL, Acree KH, et al. An outbreak of hepatitis B in a dental practice. Ann Intern Med 1981;95:133–8.

11. Carl M, Blakey DL, Francis DP, Maynard JE. Interruption of hepatitis B transmission by modification of a gynaecologist's surgical technique. Lancet 1982; i:731–3.

12. Seeff LB, Wright EC, Zimmerman HJ, et al. Type B hepatitis after needlestick exposure: prevention with hepatitis B immune globulin. Ann Intern Med 1978; 88:285–93.

13. Grady GF, Lee VA, Prince AM, et al. Hepatitis B immune globulin for accidental exposures among medical personnel: Final report of a multicenter controlled trial. J Infect Dis 1978;138:625–38.

14. Shikata T, Karasawa T, Abe K, et al. Hepatitis B e antigen and infectivity of hepatitis B virus. J Infect Dis 1977;136:571–6.

15. CDC. Update: evaluation of human T-lymphotropic virus type III/ lymphadenopathy-associated virus infection in health-care personnel—United States. MMWR 1985;34:575–8.

16. Weiss SH, Saxinger WC, Rechtman D, et al. HTLV-III infection among health care workers: association with needle-stick injuries. JAMA 1985;254:2089–93.

17. Anonymous. Needlestick transmission of HTLV-III from a patient infected in Africa. Lancet 1984;ii:1376–7.

18. Garner JS, Simmons BP. Guideline for isolation precautions in hospitals. Infect Control 1983;4:245–325.

19. Williams WW. Guideline for infection control in hospital personnel. Infect Control 1983;4:326–49.

20. CDC. Prevention of acquired immune deficiency syndrome (AIDS): report of inter-agency recommendations. MMWR 1983;32:101–3.

21. CDC. Provisional Public Health Service inter-agency recommendations for screening donated blood and plasma for antibody to the virus causing acquired immunodeficiency syndrome. MMWR 1985;34:1–5.

22. Favero MS. Sterilization, disinfection, and antisepsis in the hospital. In: Manual of Clinical Microbiology. 4th ed. Washington, D.C.: American Society for Microbiology. 1985;129–37.

23. Garner JS, Favero MS. Guideline for handwashing and hospital environmental control, 1985. Atlanta, Georgia: Centers for Disease Control, 1985. Publication no. 99-1117.

24. Kneedler JA, Dodge GH. Perioperative patient care. Boston: Blackwell Scientific Publications, 1983:210–1.
25. Martin LS, McDougal JS, Loskoski SL. Disinfection and inactivation of the human T-lymphotropic virus type III/lymphadenopathy-associated virus. J Infect Dis 1985;152:400–3.
26. Food Service Sanitation Manual 1976. DHEW publication no. (FDA) 78-2081. First printing June 1978.

Appendix C

Additional PHS Recommendations to Reduce Sexual and Drug Abuse-Related Transmission of HTLV-III/LAV

Background

Human T-lymphotropic virus type III/lymphadenopathy-associated virus (HTLV-III/LAV), the virus that causes acquired immunodeficiency syndrome (AIDS), is transmitted through sexual contact, parenteral exposure to infected blood or blood components, and perinatally from mother to fetus or neonate. In the United States, over 73% of adult AIDS patients are homosexual or bisexual men; 11% of these males also had a history of intravenous (IV) drug abuse. Seventeen percent of all adult AIDS patients were heterosexual men or women who abused IV drugs (1,2). The prevalence of HTLV-III/LAV antibody is high in certain risk groups in the United States (3,4).

Since a large proportion of seropositive asymptomatic persons have been shown to be viremic (5), all seropositive individuals, whether symptomatic or not, must be presumed capable of transmitting this infection. A repeatedly reactive serologic test for HTLV-III/LAV has important medical, as well as public health, implications for the individual and his/her health-care provider. The purpose of these recommendations is to suggest ways to facilitate identification of seropositive asymptomatic persons, both for medical evaluation and for counseling to prevent transmission.

Previous U.S. Public Health Service recommendations pertaining to sexual, IV drug abuse, and perinatal transmission of HTLV-

Source: Reprinted from *Morbidity and Mortality Weekly Report*, Vol. 35, No. 10 (March 14, 1986), pp. 152–155.

III/LAV have been published (6–8). Reduction of sexual and IV transmission of HTLV-III/LAV should be enhanced by using available serologic tests to give asymptomatic, infected individuals in high-risk groups the opportunity to know their status so they can take appropriate steps to prevent the further transmission of this virus.

Since the objective of these additional recommendations is to help interrupt transmission by encouraging testing and counseling among persons in high-risk groups, careful attention must be paid to maintaining confidentiality and to protecting records from any unauthorized disclosure. The ability of health departments to assure confidentiality—and the public confidence in that ability—are crucial to efforts to increase the number of persons requesting such testing and counseling. Without appropriate confidentiality protection, anonymous testing should be considered. Persons tested anonymously would still be offered medical evaluation and counseling.

Persons at Increased Risk of HTLV-III/LAV Infection

Persons at increased risk of HTLV-III/LAV infection include: (1) homosexual and bisexual men; (2) present or past IV drug abusers; (3) persons with clinical or laboratory evidence of infection, such as those with signs or symptoms compatible with AIDS or AIDS-related complex (ARC); (4) persons born in countries where heterosexual transmission is thought to play a major role*; (5) male or female prostitutes and their sex partners; (6) sex partners of infected persons or persons at increased risk; (7) all persons with hemophilia who have received clotting-factor products; and (8) newborn infants of high-risk or infected mothers.

Recommendations

1. Community health education programs should be aimed at members of high-risk groups to: (a) increase knowledge of AIDS; (b) facilitate behavioral changes to reduce risks of HTLV-III/LAV infection; and (c) encourage voluntary testing and counseling.
2. Counseling and voluntary serologic testing for HTLV-

---

*E.g., Haiti, central African countries.

III/LAV should be routinely offered to all persons at increased risk when they present to health-care settings. Such facilities include, but are not limited to, sexually transmitted disease clinics, clinics for treating parenteral drug abusers, and clinics for examining prostitutes.

a. Persons with a repeatedly reactive test result (see section on Test Interpretation) should receive a thorough medical evaluation, which may include history, physical examination, and appropriate laboratory studies.

b. High-risk persons with a negative test result should be counseled to reduce their risk of becoming infected by:

(1) Reducing the number of sex partners. A stable, mutually monogamous relationship with an uninfected person eliminates any new risk of sexually transmitted HTLV-III/LAV infection.

(2) Protecting themselves during sexual activity with any possibly infected person by taking appropriate precautions to prevent contact with the person's blood, semen, urine, feces, saliva, cervical secretions, or vaginal secretions. Although the efficacy of condoms in preventing infections with HTLV-III/LAV is still under study, consistent use of condoms should reduce transmission of HTLV-III/LAV by preventing exposure to semen and infected lymphocytes (9,10).

(3) For IV drug abusers, enrolling or continuing in programs to eliminate abuse of IV substances. Needles, other apparatus, and drugs must never be shared.

c. Infected persons should be counseled to prevent the further transmission of HTLV-III/LAV by:

(1) Informing prospective sex partners of his/her infection with HTLV-III/LAV, so they can take appropriate precautions. Clearly, abstention from sexual activity with another person is one option that would eliminate any risk of sexually transmitted HTLV-III/LAV infection.

(2) Protecting a partner during any sexual activity by taking appropriate precautions to prevent that individual from coming into contact with the infected person's blood, semen, urine, feces, saliva, cervical secretions, or vaginal secretions. Although the effi-

cacy of using condoms to prevent infections with
HTLV-III/LAV is still under study, consistent use of
condoms should reduce transmission of HTLV-
III/LAV by preventing exposure to semen and infected lymphocytes (*9,10*).

(3) Informing previous sex partners and any persons with
whom needles were shared of their potential exposure
to HTLV-III/LAV and encouraging them to seek
counseling/testing.

(4) For IV drug abusers, enrolling or continuing in
programs to eliminate abuse of IV substances. Needles, other apparatus, and drugs must never be
shared.

(5) Not sharing toothbrushes, razors, or other items that
could become contaminated with blood.

(6) Refraining from donating blood, plasma, body organs, other tissue, or semen.

(7) Avoiding pregnancy until more is known about the
risks of transmitting HTLV-III/LAV from mother to
fetus or newborn (*8*).

(8) Cleaning and disinfecting surfaces on which blood or
other body fluids have spilled, in accordance with
previous recommendations (*2*).

(9) Informing physicians, dentists, and other appropriate
health professionals of his/her antibody status when
seeking medical care so that the patient can be appropriately evaluated.

3. Infected patients should be encouraged to refer sex partners
or persons with whom they have shared needles to their
health-care provider for evaluation and/or testing. If patients
prefer, trained health department professionals should be
made available to assist in notifying their partners and
counseling them regarding evaluation and/or testing.

4. Persons with a negative test result should be counseled
regarding their need for continued evaluation to monitor
their infection status if they continue high-risk behavior (*8*).

5. State and local health officials should evaluate the implications of requiring the reporting of repeatedly reactive
HTLV-III/LAV antibody test results to the state health
department.

6. State or local action is appropriate on public health grounds

to regulate or close establishments where there is evidence that they facilitate high-risk behaviors, such as anonymous sexual contacts and/or intercourse with multiple partners or IV drug abuse (e.g., bathhouses, houses of prostitution, "shooting galleries").

Test Interpretation

Commercially available tests to detect antibody to HTLV-III/LAV are enzyme-linked immunosorbant assays (ELISAs) using antigens derived from disrupted HTLV-III/LAV. When the ELISA is reactive on initial testing, it is standard procedure to repeat the test on the same specimen. Repeatedly reactive tests are highly sensitive and specific for HTLV-III/LAV antibody. However, since falsely positive tests occur, and the implications of a positive test are serious, additional more specific tests (e.g., Western blot, immuno-fluorescent assay, etc.) are recommended following repeatedly reactive ELISA results, especially in low-prevalence populations. If additional more specific test results are not readily available, persons in high-risk groups with strong repeatedly reactive ELISA results can be counseled before any additional test results are received regarding their probable infection status, their need for medical follow-up, and ways to reduce further transmission of HTLV-III/LAV.

Other Considerations

State or local policies governing informing and counseling sex partners and those who share needles with persons who are HTLV-III/LAV-antibody positive will vary, depending on state and local statutes that authorize such actions. Accomplishing the objective of interrupting transmission by encouraging testing and counseling among persons in high-risk groups will depend heavily on health officials paying careful attention to maintaining confidentiality and protecting records from unauthorized disclosure.

The public health effectiveness of various approaches to counseling, sex-partner referral, and laboratory testing will require careful monitoring. The feasibility and efficacy of each of these measures should be evaluated by state and local health departments to best utilize available resources.

Developed by Center for Prevention Services and Center for Infectious Diseases, CDC, in consultation with persons from numerous other organizations and groups.

References

1. Curran JW, Morgan WM, Hardy AM, Jaffe HW, Darrow WW, Dowdle WR. The epidemiology of AIDS: current status and future prospects. Science 1985;229:1352–7.
2. CDC. Recommendations for preventing transmission of infection with human T-lymphotropic virus type III/lymphadenopathy-associated virus in the workplace. MMWR 1985;34:682–6, 691–5.
3. CDC. Update: acquired immunodeficiency syndrome in the San Francisco cohort study, 1978–1985. MMWR 1985;34:573–5.
4. CDC. Heterosexual transmission of human T-lymphotropic virus type III/lymphadenopathy-associated virus. MMWR 1985;34:561–3.
5. CDC. Provisional public health services inter-agency recommendations for screening donated blood and plasma for antibody to the virus causing acquired immunodeficiency syndrome. MMWR 1985;34:1–5.
6. CDC. Prevention of acquired immune deficiency syndrome (AIDS): report of inter-agency recommendations. MMWR 1983;32:101–4.
7. CDC. Antibodies to a retrovirus etiologically associated with acquired immunodeficiency syndrome (AIDS) in populations with increased incidences of the syndrome. MMWR 1984;33:377–9.
8. CDC. Recommendations for assisting in the prevention of perinatal transmission of human T-lymphotropic virus type III/lymphadenopathy-associated virus and acquired immunodeficiency syndrome. MMWR 1985;34:721–32.
9. Judson FN, Bodin GF, Levin MJ, Ehret JM, Masters HB. In vitro tests demonstrate condoms provide an effective barrier against chlamydia trachomatis and herpes simplex virus. Abstract in Program of the International Society for STD Research, Seattle, Washington, August 1–3, 1983:176.
10. Conant MA, Spicer DW, Smith CD. Herpes simplex virus transmission: condom studies. Sex Transm Dis 1984;11:94–5.

PHS Recommendations: Education and Foster Care of Children Infected with HTLV-III/LAV

The information and recommendations contained in this document were developed and compiled by CDC in consultation with individuals appointed by their organizations to represent the Conference of State and Territorial Epidemiologists, the Association of State and Territorial Health Officers, the National Association of County Health Officers, the Division of Maternal and Child Health (Health Resources and Services Administration), the National Association for Elementary School Principals, the National Association of State School Nurse Consultants, the National Congress of Parents and Teachers, and the Children's Aid Society. The consultants also included the mother of a child with acquired immunodeficiency syndrome (AIDS), a legal advisor to a state education department, and several pediatricians who are experts in the field of pediatric AIDS. This document is made available to assist state and local health and education departments in developing guidelines for their particular situations and locations.

These recommendations apply to all children known to be infected with human T-lymphotropic virus type III/lymphadenopathy-associated virus (HTLV-III/LAV). This includes children with AIDS as defined for reporting purposes (Table 1); children who are diagnosed by their physicians as having an illness due to infection with HTLV-III/LAV but who do not meet the case definition; and children who are asymptomatic but have virologic or serologic evidence of infection with HTLV-III/LAV. These recommendations

Source: Reprinted from *Morbidity and Mortality Weekly Report*, Vol. 34 (Aug. 30, 1985), pp. 517–521.

do not apply to siblings of infected children unless they are also infected.

Background

The Scope of the Problem   As of August 20, 1985, 183 of the 12,599 reported cases of AIDS in the United States were among children under 18 years of age. This number is expected to double in the next year. Children with AIDS have been reported from 23 states, the District of Columbia, and Puerto Rico, with 75% residing in New York, California, Florida, and New Jersey.

The 183 AIDS patients reported to CDC represent only the most severe form of HTLV-III/LAV infection, i.e., those children who develop opportunistic infections or malignancies (Table 1). As in adults with HTLV-III/LAV infection, many infected children may have milder illness or may be asymptomatic.

TABLE 1. Provisional Case Definition for Acquired Immuno-deficiency Syndrome (AIDS) Surveillance of Children

For the limited purposes of epidemiologic surveillance, CDC defines a case of pediatric acquired immunodeficiency syndrome (AIDS) as a child who has had:
1. A reliably diagnosed disease at least moderately indicative of underlying cellular immunodeficiency, and
2. No known cause of underlying cellular immunodeficiency or any other reduced resistance reported to be associated with that disease.

The diseases accepted as sufficiently indicative of underlying cellular immunodeficiency are the same as those used in defining AIDS in adults. In the absence of these opportunistic diseases, a histologically confirmed diagnosis of chronic lymphoid interstitial pneumonitis will be considered indicative of AIDS unless test(s) for HTLV-III/LAV are negative. Congenital infections, e.g., toxoplasmosis or herpes simplex virus infection in the first month after birth or cytomegalovirus infection in the first 6 months after birth must be excluded.

Specific conditions that must be excluded in a child are:
1. Primary immunodeficiency diseases—severe combined immunode-ficiency, DiGeorge syndrome, Wiskott-Aldrich syndrome, ataxia-telangiectasia, graft versus host disease, neutropenia, neutrophil function abnormality, agammaglobulinemia, or hypogammaglob-ulinemia with raised IgM.
2. Secondary immunodeficiency associated with immunosuppressive therapy, lymphoreticular malignancy, or starvation.

Legal Issues   Among the legal issues to be considered in forming guidelines for the education and foster care of HTLV-III/LAV-infected children are the civil rights aspects of public school attendance, the protections for handicapped children under 20 U.S.C. 1401 et seq. and 29 U.S.C. 794, the confidentiality of a student's school record under state laws and under 20 U.S.C. 1232g, and employee right-to-know statutes for public employees in some states.

Confidentiality Issues   The diagnosis of AIDS or associated illnesses evokes much fear from others in contact with the patient and may evoke suspicion of life styles that may not be acceptable to some persons. Parents of HTLV-III/LAV-infected children should be aware of the potential for social isolation should the child's condition become known to others in the care or educational setting. School, day-care, and social service personnel and others involved in educating and caring for these children should be sensitive to the need for confidentiality and the right to privacy in these cases.

Assessment of Risks

Risk Factors for Acquiring HTLV-III/LAV Infection and Transmission   In adults and adolescents, HTLV-III/LAV is transmitted primarily through sexual contact (homosexual or heterosexual) and through parenteral exposure to infected blood or blood products. HTLV-III/LAV has been isolated from blood, semen, saliva, and tears but transmission has not been documented from saliva and tears. Adults at increased risk for acquiring HTLV-III/LAV include homosexual/bisexual men, intravenous drug abusers, persons transfused with contaminated blood or blood products, and sexual contacts of persons with HTLV-III/LAV infection or in groups at increased risk for infection.

The majority of infected children acquire the virus from their infected mothers in the perinatal period (1–4). In utero or intrapartum transmission are likely, and one child reported from Australia apparently acquired the virus postnatally, possibly from ingestion of breast milk (5). Children may also become infected through transfusion of blood or blood products that contain the virus. Seventy percent of the pediatric cases reported to CDC occurred among children whose parent had AIDS or was a member of a group at increased risk of acquiring HTLV-III/LAV infection; 20% of the cases occurred among children who had received blood or blood products; and for 10%, investigations are incomplete.

Risk of Transmission in the School, Day-Care or Foster-Care Setting None of the identified cases of HTLV-III/LAV infection in the United States are known to have been transmitted in the school, day-care, or foster-care setting or through other casual person-to-person contact. Other than the sexual partners of HTLV-III/LAV-infected patients and infants born to infected mothers, none of the family members of the over 12,000 AIDS patients reported to CDC have been reported to have AIDS. Six studies of family members of patients with HTLV-III/LAV infection have failed to demonstrate HTLV-III/LAV transmission to adults who were not sexual contacts of the infected patients or to older children who were not likely at risk from perinatal transmission (6–11).

Based on current evidence, casual person-to-person contact as would occur among schoolchildren appears to pose no risk. However, studies of the risk of transmission through contact between younger children and neurologically handicapped children who lack control of their body secretions are very limited. Based on experience with other communicable diseases, a theoretical potential for transmission would be greatest among these children. It should be emphasized that any theoretical transmission would most likely involve exposure of open skin lesions or mucous membranes to blood and possibly other body fluids of an infected person.

Risks to the Child with HTLV-III/LAV Infection HTLV-III/LAV infection may result in immunodeficiency. Such children may have a greater risk of encountering infectious agents in a school or day-care setting than at home. Foster homes with multiple children may also increase the risk. In addition, younger children and neurologically handicapped children who may display behaviors such as mouthing of toys would be expected to be at greater risk for acquiring infections. Immunodepressed children are also at greater risk of suffering severe complications from such infections as chickenpox, cytomegalovirus, tuberculosis, herpes simplex, and measles. Assessment of the risk to the immunodepressed child is best made by the child's physician who is aware of the child's immune status. The risk of acquiring some infections, such as chickenpox, may be reduced by prompt use of specific immune globulin following a known exposure.

Recommendations

1. Decisions regarding the type of educational and care setting for HTLV-III/LAV-infected children should be based on the behavior, neurologic development, and physical condition of the child and the expected type of interaction with others in that setting. These decisions are best made using the team approach including the child's physician, public health personnel, the child's parent or guardian, and personnel associated with the proposed care or educational setting. In each case, risks and benefits to both the infected child and to others in the setting should be weighed.

2. For most infected school-aged children, the benefits of an unrestricted setting would outweigh the risks of their acquiring potentially harmful infections in the setting and the apparent non-existent risk of transmission of HTLV-III/LAV. These children should be allowed to attend school and after-school day-care and to be placed in a foster home in an unrestricted setting.

3. For the infected preschool-aged child and for some neurologically handicapped children who lack control of their body secretions or who display behavior, such as biting, and those children who have uncoverable, oozing lesions, a more restricted environment is advisable until more is known about transmission in these settings. Children infected with HTLV-III/LAV should be cared for and educated in settings that minimize exposure of other children to blood or body fluids.

4. Care involving exposure to the infected child's body fluids and excrement, such as feeding and diaper changing, should be performed by persons who are aware of the child's HTLV-III/LAV infection and the modes of possible transmission. In any setting involving an HTLV-III/LAV-infected person, good handwashing after exposure to blood and body fluids and before caring for another child should be observed, and gloves should be worn if open lesions are present on the caretaker's hands. Any open lesions on the infected person should also be covered.

5. Because other infections in addition to HTLV-III/LAV can be present in blood or body fluids, all schools and day-care facilities, regardless of whether children with HTLV-III/LAV infection are attending, should adopt routine procedures for handling blood or body fluids. Soiled surfaces should be promptly cleaned with disinfectants, such as household bleach (diluted 1 part bleach to 10 parts water). Disposable towels or tissues should be used whenever

possible, and mops should be rinsed in the disinfectant. Those who are cleaning should avoid exposure of open skin lesions or mucous membranes to the blood or body fluids.

6. The hygienic practices of children with HTLV-III/LAV infection may improve as the child matures. Alternatively, the hygienic practices may deteriorate if the child's condition worsens. Evaluation to assess the need for a restricted environment should be performed regularly.

7. Physicians caring for children born to mothers with AIDS or at increased risk of acquiring HTLV-III/LAV infection should consider testing the children for evidence of HTLV-III/LAV infection for medical reasons. For example, vaccination of infected children with live virus vaccines, such as the measles–mumps–rubella vaccine (MMR), may be hazardous. These children also need to be followed closely for problems with growth and development and given prompt and aggressive therapy for infections and exposure to potentially lethal infections, such as varicella. In the event that an antiviral agent or other therapy for HTLV-III/LAV infection becomes available, these children should be considered for such therapy. Knowledge that a child is infected will allow parents and other caretakers to take precautions when exposed to the blood and body fluids of the child.

8. Adoption and foster-care agencies should consider adding HTLV-III/LAV screening to their routine medical evaluations of children at increased risk of infection before placement in the foster or adoptive home, since these parents must make decisions regarding the medical care of the child and must consider the possible social and psychological effects on their families.

9. Mandatory screening as a condition for school entry is not warranted based on available data.

10. Persons involved in the care and education of HTLV-III/LAV-infected children should respect the child's right to privacy, including maintaining confidential records. The number of personnel who are aware of the child's condition should be kept at a minimum needed to assure proper care of the child and to detect situations where the potential for transmission may increase (e.g., bleeding injury).

11. All educational and public health departments, regardless of whether HTLV-III/LAV-infected children are involved, are strongly encouraged to inform parents, children, and educators regarding HTLV-III/LAV and its transmission. Such education would greatly

assist efforts to provide the best care and education for infected children while minimizing the risk of transmission to others.

References

1. Scott GB, Buck BE, Leterman JG, Bloom FL, Parks WP. Acquired immunodeficiency syndrome in infants. N Engl J Med 1984;310:76–81.
2. Thomas PA, Jaffe HW, Spira TJ, Reiss R,Guerrero IC, Auerbach D. Unexplained immunodeficiency in children. A surveillance report. JAMA 1984;252:639–44.
3. Rubinstein A, Sicklick M, Gupta A, et al. Acquired immunodeficiency with reversed T4/T8 ratios in infants born to promiscuous and drug-addicted mothers. JAMA 1983;249:2350–6.
4. Oleske J, Minnefor A, Cooper R Jr, et al. Immune deficiency syndrome in children. JAMA 1983;249:2345–9.
5. Ziegler JB, Cooper DA, Johnson RO, Gold J. Postnatal transmission of AIDS-associated retrovirus from mother to infant. Lancet 1985;i:896–8.
6. CDC. Unpublished data.
7. Kaplan JE, Oleske JM, Getchell JP, et al. Evidence against transmission of HTLV-III/LAV in families of children with AIDS. Pediatric Infectious Disease (in press).
8. Lewin EB, Zack R, Ayodele A. Communicability of AIDS in a foster care setting. International Conference on Acquired Immunodeficiency Syndrome (AIDS), Atlanta, Georgia, April 1985.
9. Thomas PA, Lubin K, Enlow RW, Getchell J. Comparison of HTLV-III serology, T-cell levels, and general health status of children whose mothers have AIDS with children of healthy inner city mothers in New York. International Conference on Acquired Immunodeficiency Syndrome (AIDS), Atlanta, Georgia, April 1985.
10. Fischl MA, Dickinson G, Scott G, Klimas N, Fletcher M, Parks W. Evaluation of household contacts of adult patients with the acquired immunodeficiency syndrome. International Conference on Acquired Immunodeficiency Syndrome (AIDS), Atlanta, Georgia, April 1985.
11. Friedland GH, Saltzman BR, Rogers MF, et al. Lack of household transmission of HTLV-III infection. EIS Conference, Atlanta, Georgia, April 1985.

Appendix E

Organizations to Contact for Information on AIDS

Following is a list of national and selected local service organizations that offer information of various types (e.g., recorded messages, printed material, M.D. referrals, legal information, and statistics) on AIDS.*

NATIONAL

Centers for Disease Control
Hotline: 1-800-342-AIDS (Recorded information)
            1-800-447-AIDS (Specific questions)
In Atlanta: (404) 329-3534 (Printed material)
            (404) 329-1290 (Recorded information)
            (404) 329-1295 (Specific questions)

National Institute of Allergy and Infectious Diseases
Office of Research Reporting and Public Response
(301) 496-5717

Public Health Service
1-800-342-AIDS (Recorded information)
1-800-447-AIDS (Specific questions)

*Source: Adapted, with permission, from Journal of the American Medical Association, Vol. 254, No. 18 (Nov. 8, 1985), pp. 2522–2523. Copyright 1985, American Medical Association. See JAMA for a more complete listing of local organizations.

American Red Cross
AIDS Public Education Program
Contact local chapter for information.

American Association of Physicians for Human Rights
    (M.D. referrals)
P.O. Box 14366
San Francisco, CA 94114
(415) 673-3189

Public Health Service
Preventive Health Services Administration (Statistics on AIDS)
(202) 673-3525

National Gay and Lesbian Task Force
1517 U St., NW
Washington, DC 20009
(202) 332-6483
    Fund for Human Dignity
    (212) 741-5800 (Educational material)
    National Gay and Lesbian Crisis Line
    1-800-221-7044 (Crisis counseling)

National Hemophilia Foundation
Soho Building
110 Greene Street, Room 406
New York, NY 10012
(212) 219-8180

National Lesbian and Gay Health Foundation (Health care referrals)
P.O. Box 65472
Washington, DC 20035
(202) 797-3708
    National Association of People with AIDS
    (202) 483-7979

LOCAL

CALIFORNIA

California Department of Health Services
AIDS Activities
P.O. Box 160146
Sacramento, CA 95816-0146
1-800-367-2437 (Northern California hotline)
1-800-922-2437 (Southern California hotline)
TTY number: (415) 864-6606

AIDS Project/Los Angeles
837 No. Cole Street, Suite 3
Los Angeles, CA 90038
(213) 876-8951 (Administration)
(213) 876-9072 (Hotline)

San Diego AIDS Project
4304 3rd Ave.
P.O. Box 81082
San Diego, CA 92138
(619) 543-0300

San Francisco AIDS Foundation
333 Valencia Street, Fourth Floor
San Francisco, CA 94103
(415) 863-AIDS (Hotline)

DISTRICT OF COLUMBIA

AIDS Action Project
Whitman-Walker Clinic
2335 18th Street, NW
Washington, DC 20009
(202) 332-AIDS
  AIDS Program
  (202) 332-5939 (Information on support groups)

St. Francis Center (Grief and bereavement counseling)
2201 P St., NW
Washington, DC 20037
(202) 234-5613

FLORIDA

AIDS Education Project (Counseling, education, etc.)
P.O. Box 4073
Key West, FL 33041
(305) 294-8302

Health Crisis Network (Counseling)
P.O. Box 52-1546
Miami, FL 33152
(305) 634-4636

NEW YORK

Gay Men's Health Crisis
Box 274
132 West 24th Street
New York, NY 10011
(212) 807-6655 (Direct advice)
(212) 807-7517 (Education)

AIDS Resource Center, Inc. (Residential treatment; bereavement
    counseling)
P.O. Box 792
Chelsea Street Station
New York, NY 10011
(212) 206-1414

HTLV-III Hotline
N.Y. City Department of Health
c/o Office of Public Health Education
125 Worth Street
New York, NY 10013
(212) 566-7103 (Literature)
(212) 566-8290 (Speakers, public health information)
(718) 485-8111 (Hotline)

Suggested Readings

"AIDS: A time bomb at hospitals' door." *Hospitals* (Jan. 5, 1986), pp. 54–61.

Bayer, Ronald, and Gerald Oppenheimer. "AIDS in the Workplace: The Ethical Ramifications." *Business and Health* (Jan./Feb. 1986), pp. 30–34.

DeVita, Vincent T., Jr., Samuel Hellman, and Steven A. Rosenberg, eds. *AIDS: Etiology, Diagnosis, Treatment, and Prevention.* Philadelphia: Lippincott, 1985.

Gallin, John I., and Anthony S. Fauci, eds. *Acquired Immunodeficiency Syndrome (AIDS).* Advances in Host Defense Mechanisms, Vol. 5. New York: Raven Press, 1985.

International Conference on Acquired Immunodeficiency Syndrome, 14–17 April 1985, Atlanta, Georgia—selected papers. *Annals of Internal Medicine,* Vol. 103, No. 5 (November 1985), pp. 653–781.

Johnson, Richard T., and Justin C. McArthur. "AIDS and the Brain." *Trends in Neuroscience,* Vol. 9, No. 3 (March 1986), pp. 91–94.

Jonsen, Albert R., Molly Cooke, and Barbara A. Koenig. "AIDS and Ethics." *Issues in Science and Technology,* Vol. 2, No. 2 (Winter 1986), pp. 56–65.

Kanki, Phyllis J., Francis Barin, Souleyman M'Boup, Jonathan S. Allan, Jean Loup Romet-Lemonne, Richard Marlink, Mary Francis McLane, Tun-Hou Lee, Brigitte Arbeille, François Denis, and M. Essex. "New Human T-lymphotropic Retrovirus Related to Simian T-lymphotropic Virus Type-III (STLV-III$_{AGM}$)." *Science,* Vol. 232, No. 4747 (April 11, 1986), pp. 238–243.

Lee, Philip R. "AIDS: Allocating Resources for Research and Patient Care." *Issues in Science and Technology*, Vol. 2, No. 2 (Winter 1986), pp. 66–73.

Levine, Carol, and Joyce Bermel, eds. *AIDS: The Emerging Ethical Dilemmas*. Hastings Center Report Special Supplement. Vol. 15, No. 4 (August 1985). Hastings-on-Hudson, N.Y.: Hastings Center.

Nichols, Stuart E., and David G. Ostrow, eds. *Psychiatric Implications of Acquired Immune Deficiency Syndrome*. Washington, D.C.: American Psychiatric Press, 1984.

Osborn, June E. "The AIDS Epidemic: An Overview of the Science." *Issues in Science and Technology*, Vol. 2, No. 2 (Winter 1986), pp. 40–55.

"A Review of State and Local Government Initiatives Affecting AIDS." Washington, D.C.: Intergovernmental Health Policy Project at the George Washington University, November 1985.

"Review of the Public Health Service's Response to AIDS. A Technical Memorandum." OTA-TM-H-24. Washington, D.C.: Office of Technology Assessment, Congress of the United States, February 1985.

Glossary

ACQUIRED IMMUNE DEFICIENCY SYNDROME (AIDS)   A severe late manifestation of infection with the virus HTLV-III/LAV. The virus destroys or incapacitates important components of the human immune system. Persons with this disease develop infections caused by microorganisms that usually do not produce infections in persons with normal immunity.

AIDS-RELATED COMPLEX (ARC)   A variety of chronic symptoms and physical findings that occur in some persons who are infected with HTLV-III/LAV, but whose conditions do not meet the Centers for Disease Control's definition of AIDS. Symptoms may include chronic swollen glands, recurrent fevers, unintentional weight loss, chronic diarrhea, lethargy, minor alterations of the immune system (less severe than those that occur in AIDS), and oral thrush. ARC may or may not develop into AIDS.

ANTIBODY   A protein in the blood produced in response to exposure to specific foreign molecules. Antibodies neutralize toxins and interact with other components of the immune system to eliminate infectious microorganisms from the body.

ANTIGEN   A substance that stimulates the production of antibodies.

ARV (AIDS-ASSOCIATED RETROVIRUS)   Name given by researchers at the University of California at San Francisco to isolates of the retrovirus that causes AIDS. (*See also* HTLV-III/LAV.)

AUTOLOGOUS TRANSFUSION   A blood transfusion in which the patient receives his or her own blood, donated several weeks before elective surgery.

B LYMPHOCYTE (OR B CELL)   A type of white blood cell that produces antibody in response to stimulation by an antigen.

CANDIDA ALBICANS   A yeastlike fungus that causes whitish sores in the mouth. The infection is called candidiasis, or, more commonly, thrush. In AIDS patients, candidiasis often extends into the esophagus.

CELL-MEDIATED IMMUNITY   A defense mechanism involving the coordinated activity of two subpopulations of T lymphocytes, helper T cells and killer T cells. Helper T cells produce a variety of substances that stimulate and regulate other participants in the immune response. Killer T lymphocytes destroy cells in the body that are infected with viruses or other microorganisms.

COFACTOR   A factor other than the basic causative agent of a disease that increases the likelihood of developing that disease. Cofactors may include the presence of other microorganisms or psychosocial factors, such as stress.

CRYPTOSPORIDIUM   A protozoan parasite that causes severe, protracted diarrhea. In persons with a normal immune system, the diarrhea is self-limited and lasts one to two weeks. In AIDS patients, the diarrhea often becomes chronic and may lead to severe malnutrition.

CYTOMEGALOVIRUS (CMV)   A virus that belongs to the herpesvirus group. Prior to the appearance of AIDS, it was most commonly associated with a severe congenital infection of infants and with life-threatening infections in patients who had undergone bone marrow transplants and other procedures requiring suppression of the immune system. It rarely causes disease in healthy adults. In AIDS patients, CMV may produce pneumonia, as well as inflammation of the retina, liver, kidneys, and colon.

DNA (DEOXYRIBONUCLEIC ACID)   A nucleic acid found chiefly in the nucleus of living cells that is responsible for transmitting hereditary characteristics.

ELISA   An acronym for "enzyme-linked immunosorbent assay," a test used to detect antibodies against the virus HTLV-III/LAV in blood samples.

ENCEPHALITIS   Inflammation of the brain.

ENCEPHALOPATHY   Any degenerative disease of the brain.

ENZYME   Any of a group of proteins produced by living cells that mediate and promote the chemical processes of life without themselves being altered or destroyed.

EPSTEIN-BARR VIRUS   A member of the herpes group of viruses and the principal cause of infectious mononucleosis in young adults.

It also has been implicated as a causal factor in the development of Burkitt's lymphoma in Africa.

GENOME   The genetic endowment of an organism.

HEMOGLOBIN   The protein found in red blood cells that contains iron and carries oxygen.

HEMOPHILIA   A rare, hereditary bleeding disorder of males, inherited through the mother, caused by a deficiency in the ability to make one or more blood–clotting proteins.

HERPES SIMPLEX   An acute disease caused by herpes simplex viruses types 1 and 2. Groups of watery blisters, often painful, form on the skin and mucous membranes, especially the borders of the lips (cold sores) or the mucous surface of the genitals.

HERPESVIRUS GROUP   A group of viruses that includes the herpes simplex viruses, the varicella-zoster virus (the cause of chicken pox and shingles), cytomegalovirus, and Epstein-Barr virus.

HTLV-III (HUMAN T-CELL LYMPHOTROPIC VIRUS, TYPE III)   The name given by researchers at the National Cancer Institute to isolates of the retrovirus that causes AIDS.

HTLV-III/LAV   The name used in this book for the retrovirus that causes AIDS and related conditions. (*See also* HTLV-III and LAV.)

HUMORAL IMMUNITY   The human defense mechanism that involves the production of antibodies.

IMMUNE SYSTEM   The natural system of defense mechanisms, in which specialized cells and proteins in the blood and other body fluids work together to eliminate disease-producing microorganisms and other foreign substances.

INTERFERONS   A class of proteins important in immune function and known to inhibit certain viral infections.

INTERLEUKIN-2 (IL-2)   A substance produced by T lymphocytes that stimulates other T lymphocytes to proliferate. Also known as T-cell growth factor.

INTERSTITIAL PNEUMONITIS   Localized acute inflammation of the lung. Interstitial pneumonitis persisting for more than two months in a child (under 13 years of age) is indicative of AIDS unless another cause is identified or tests for HTLV-III/LAV are negative.

INTRAVENOUS   Injected into or delivered through a needle in a vein.

KAPOSI'S SARCOMA (KS)   A cancer or tumor of the blood vessel walls. It usually appears as blue-violet to brownish skin blotches or bumps. Before the appearance of AIDS, it was rare in the United States and Europe, where it occurred primarily in men over age 50 or 60, usually of Mediterranean origin. AIDS-associated Kaposi's sarcoma is much more aggressive than the earlier form of the disease.

LAV (LYMPHADENOPATHY-ASSOCIATED VIRUS)   The name given by French researchers to the first reported isolate of the retrovirus now known to cause AIDS. This retrovirus was recovered from a person with lymphadenopathy (enlarged lymph nodes) who also was in a group at high risk of AIDS. (*See also* HTLV-III and HTLV-III/LAV.)

LENTIVIRUSES   A subfamily of retroviruses that includes the visna viruses of sheep, the equine infectious anemia virus of horses, and the caprine arthritis-encephalitis virus of goats. Most researchers believe that HTLV-III/LAV, the cause of AIDS, also belongs to this subfamily. The animal lentiviruses produce diverse chronic diseases in their natural hosts, but all cause encephalitis. The diseases are characterized by erratic relapses and remissions. The visna viruses cause a chronic interstitial pneumonitis similar to that seen in AIDS virus infections in infants. Lentiviruses persist in the body by evading natural defense mechanisms; the chronic carrier state—in which infected animals do not get sick themselves but can transmit the virus to other animals—is common.

LYMPHADENOPATHY SYNDROME   A condition characterized by persistent (more than three months), generalized swollen glands in the absence of any current illness or drug use known to cause such symptoms.

MONOCYTE   A phagocytic white blood cell that engulfs and destroys bacteria and other disease-producing microorganisms. It produces interleukin-1, a substance that activates T lymphocytes in the presence of antigen.

MUTATION   A change in the genetic material of a cell or a virus that may lead to a change in the structure or function of a protein.

MYCOBACTERIUM AVIUM-INTRACELLULARE   A bacterium related to the organism that causes tuberculosis in humans, rarely seen by physicians prior to the appearance of AIDS. In AIDS patients, it may cause a disseminated disease that responds poorly to therapy.

ONCOVIRUSES   A subfamily of retroviruses that includes tumor-causing agents such as the Rous sarcoma virus and the bovine leukemia virus.

OPPORTUNISTIC INFECTION   An infection caused by a microorganism that rarely causes disease in persons with normal defense mechanisms.

PHAGOCYTE   A white blood cell that binds to, engulfs, and destroys microorganisms, damaged cells, and foreign particles.

PNEUMOCYSTIS CARINII PNEUMONIA   The most common life-threatening opportunistic infection diagnosed in AIDS patients. It is caused by the parasite *Pneumocystis carinii*.

PROVIRUS   A copy of the genetic information of an animal virus that is integrated into the DNA of an infected cell. Copies of the provirus are passed on to each of the infected cell's daughter cells.

RETROVIRUS   A class of viruses that contain the genetic material RNA and that have the capability to copy this RNA into DNA inside an infected cell. The resulting DNA is incorporated into the genetic structure of the cell in the form of a provirus.

REVERSE TRANSCRIPTASE   An enzyme produced by retroviruses that allows them to produce a DNA copy of their RNA. This is the first step in the virus's natural cycle of reproduction.

RNA (RIBONUCLEIC ACID)   A nucleic acid associated with the control of chemical activities inside a cell. One type of RNA transfers information from the cell's DNA to the protein-forming system of a cell outside the nucleus. Some viruses carry RNA instead of the more familiar genetic material DNA.

SEROPOSITIVE   A condition in which antibodies to a particular disease-producing organism are found in the blood. The presence of antibodies indicates that a person has been exposed to the organism, but does not distinguish between an active infection and a past infection. (Researchers believe that most persons with antibodies against HTLV-III/LAV carry active virus particles and therefore should be considered infectious to others through sexual practices that involve an exchange of body fluids, through sharing of intravenous needles, and, for women, through transmission to an unborn or breastfed child.)

SUBUNIT VACCINE   A vaccine that contains only portions of a surface molecule of a disease-producing microorganism.

SYNDROME   A pattern of symptoms and signs, appearing one by one or simultaneously, that together characterize a particular disease or disorder.

T LYMPHOCYTE (OR T CELL)   A white blood cell that matures in the thymus gland. Subsets of T cells have a variety of specialized functions within the immune system. (*See also* cell-mediated immunity and T4 lymphocyte.)

T4 LYMPHOCYTE (OR T4 CELL)   A subset of T lymphocytes that act as master regulators of the human immune system. These cells appear to be the primary targets of the virus HTLV–III/LAV.

TOXOPLASMA GONDII   A protozoan parasite that is one of the most common causes of inflammation of the brain in AIDS patients. The infection is called toxoplasmosis.

WESTERN BLOT TECHNIQUE   A test that involves the identification of antibodies against specific protein molecules. This test is believed to be more specific than the ELISA in detecting HTLV-III/LAV antibodies in blood samples; it is also more difficult to perform and considerably more expensive. Western blot analysis is used by some laboratories as a confirmatory test on samples found to be repeatably reactive on the ELISA.

Contributors and Acknowledgments

The 1985 annual meeting of the Institute of Medicine focused on AIDS at the suggestion of Frederick C. Robbins, then president of the IOM. Chaired by Philip Leder, John Emory Andrus Professor, and chairman, Department of Genetics, Harvard Medical School, the meeting was planned and carried out under the skillful direction of Enriqueta C. Bond, director of IOM's Division of Health Promotion and Disease Prevention. The challenging task of writing the book based on the meeting was performed by Eve K. Nichols.

Speakers who addressed the meeting also graciously cooperated throughout the preparation of the book:

LEWELLYS F. BARKER, Senior Vice President, American Red Cross

RONALD BAYER, Associate for Policy Studies, The Hastings Center

BRETT J. CASSENS, Immediate Past President, American Association of Physicians for Human Rights

JAMES W. CURRAN, Chief, AIDS Branch, Division of Viral Diseases, Center for Infectious Disease, Centers for Disease Control

ANTHONY S. FAUCI, Director, National Institute of Allergy and Infectious Diseases, National Institutes of Health

SHERVERT FRAZIER, Director, National Institute of Mental Health; Alcohol, Drug Abuse, and Mental Health Administration

ROBERT C. GALLO, Chief, Laboratory of Tumor Cell Biology, National Cancer Institute, National Institutes of Health

RICHARD T. JOHNSON, Dwight D. Eisenhower Professor of Neurology and Professor of Microbiology, Johns Hopkins University School of Medicine

PHILIP R. LEE, Director, Institute for Health Policy Studies,
    University of California, San Francisco
LUC MONTAGNIER, Head, Viral Oncology Unit, Institut Pasteur,
    Paris
JUNE E. OSBORN, Dean, School of Public Health, University of
    Michigan
FREDERICK C. ROBBINS, then-President, Institute of Medicine
MERVYN F. SILVERMAN, Consultant and Former Director of
    Health, San Francisco

The writing of the manuscript was made possible by a grant
from Hoffman-La Roche, Inc., and the National Research Council
Fund, a pool of private, discretionary, nonfederal funds used to
support programs initiated by the National Academy of Sciences
that are concerned with national issues in which science and technology figure significantly.

The planning, development, and production of this volume
were overseen by the National Academy Press, publisher for the
Institute of Medicine, the National Academy of Sciences, the National Academy of Engineering, and the National Research Council.
The project editor was Dorothy Sawicki.

Index

AAPHR (American Association of Physicians for Human Rights), 92, 125, 126
Acupuncture, 37, 167
Adjustment to AIDS, 120–121, 123
Adoption agencies, 183
Adult T-cell leukemia (ATL) syndrome, 65
Africa
  Burkitt's lymphoma in, 54
  cryptococcal meningitis in, 45
  incidence in, 16–18, 39
  Kaposi's sarcoma in, 16–17, 50
AIDS, definitions of, 44–45, 149–154
AIDS-associated retrovirus (ARV), 67, 68
AIDS-related complex (ARC)
  defined, 19
  lymphadenopathy syndrome and, 51–53
  pattern of symptoms in, 19–20, 52
  progression to AIDS, 22, 52–53, 173
  psychosocial impact of, 123–124
Airline attendants, 168
Alpha interferon, 49, 107

American Association of Physicians for Human Rights (AAPHR), 92, 125, 126
Amyl nitrite, 60, 97
Anal intercourse, 11, 60
Anger
  in AIDS patients, 120, 123
  in ARC patients, 124
Angioimmunoblastic lymphadenopathy, 154
Animal models, 115
Ansamycin, 110
Antibodies
  in AIDS, 82–83
  to HTLV-III/LAV, 85, 88, 114–115
  in immune response, 75, 76–78
  to STLV-III, 116
Antibody tests, 20–21, 33–38. See also Testing
Antigen
  defined, 75
  immune response to, 75–78
Antimoniotungstate, 109–110
Anxiety, 125
ARC. See AIDS-related complex (ARC)
ARV (AIDS-associated retrovirus), 67, 68
Azidothymidine, 112–113

Bacterial infections, 43, 151. *See also* Opportunistic infections
Barbers, 100, 167
Barker, Lewellys F., 40
Bartenders, 155, 168
Bathhouses, 98, 140–141,176
Bayer, Ronald, 131, 146
Bisexual men, 18, 27, 99. *See also* Homosexual men
Blacks, incidence in, 14
Bleach, household, 11, 37, 161, 166, 168
Blindness, 46
Blood, transmission in, 155–168. *See also* Blood donors; Blood transfusions
Blood bank technologists. *See* Health care personnel
Blood donors
  designated, 101
  high-risk, 67–68
  notification of, 33–35, 36, 37
  screening of, 12, 32–38
  transmission to, misconceptions about, 101
Blood transfusions
  in children, 38–39, 180–181
  in foreign countries, 19
  incidence from, 3, 13, 32, 38–39
  risk reduction in, 32–39
B lymphocytes
  in AIDS, 80, 82–83, 87
  function of, 75, 76–78
Bone marrow transplants, 110
Brain disease
  in definition of AIDS, 44, 58, 151
  from HTLV-III/LAV, 54–56, 85–87, 88
  psychosocial impact of, 123
  signs of, 54–56
Breast feeding, 12, 30, 180
Broder, Samuel, 112

Burkitt's lymphoma, 54, 152

Cancer, 58, 151, 154. *See also* Kaposi's sarcoma; Lymphomas
Candidiasis, 47, 52, 150, 151–152
Caprine arthritis-encephalitis virus, 72
Cardiopulmonary resuscitation (CPR), 100, 160, 162
Cassens, Brett J., 117, 125, 131, 146
Casual contact, lack of transmission from, 10, 11, 156
Caterers, 155, 168
Cell-mediated immunity, 75–76, 78, 79
Chemotherapy, for Kaposi's sarcoma, 50
Children
  blood transfusions in, 38–39
  diagnosis in, 56, 58, 152, 154
  findings in, 57
  foster care for, 178–184
  incidence in, 29
  at risk, 29–30, 38–39, 56, 180–181
  in school setting, 99–100, 122, 178–184
  transmission to, 11, 12, 29–30, 180–181
  vaccine intolerance in, 57
Chimpanzees, infected by HTLV-III/LAV, 115
Chiropractors. *See* Health care personnel
Civil rights issues, 8, 139–145, 180
Classroom, AIDS in, 99–100, 122, 178–184
Cleaning
  of dishes, 166
  of laundry, 166

Cleaning *(cont)*
of spills, 161, 166, 183
CMV. *See* Cytomegalovirus
(CMV)
Cofactors, 22, 52, 97, 126
Condoms, 12, 37, 102, 174–175
Confidentiality
in AIDS research, 133
and anonymous testing, 125–
126, 173
for children, 180, 183
and mandatory reporting, 8,
98–99, 125–126
Public Health Service policy
on, 36, 95, 173, 176
Consent, informed, 123
Construction sites, 168
Contact tracing, 8, 98–99, 140,
176
Cooks, 155, 168
Corticosteroid therapy, 153
Cosmetologists, 167
Costs
economic, 3–4
for educational programs, 136–
137
hospital, 23, 134, 138–139
research, 136, 137
responsibility for, 7–8, 135–
138
Coughing, 10
Counseling
for AIDS patients, 120, 122
for high-risk individuals, 95–
97, 173–175
information on, 185–188
CPR (cardiopulmonary resuscitation), 100, 160, 162
Cryptococcal meningitis, 45
Cryptococcosis, 151
Cryptosporidium infection, 44, 48,
150
Curran, James W., 23–24, 40,
58, 117

Cyclosporin A, 110
Cytomegalovirus (CMV)
and B lymphocytes, 83
in definition of AIDS, 151, 154
and Kaposi's sarcoma, 46, 50
infection with, 46–47
treatment of, 47
Cytotoxic T lymphocytes, 75,
76, 78, 79, 85

Daniel, M. D., 71
Day care facilities, 100, 122, 181
Death rate, 2, 14, 42
De Clercq, Erik, 107
Decontamination, of surgical in-
struments, 165. *See also*
Sterilization, of instruments
Definitions, of AIDS, 44–45,
149–154
Dementia
CAT scan, 55
from HTLV-III/LAV, 71, 86
psychosocial impact of, 123,
130
Denial, 119–120
Dental care personnel. *See also*
Health care personnel
informing, 37
precautions for, 31–32
sterilization procedures for, 32,
165–166
Depression, 120, 123
Dermatitis, weeping, 164, 167
Designated donors, 101
Des Jarlais, Don C., 94
Diagnosis, 44–45, 149–154
in children, 56, 58, 152, 154
Dialysis personnel. *See* Health
care personnel
Diaper changing, 182
Discrimination
against AIDS patients, 121–122
education and, 7

Discrimination (*cont*)
   against homosexuals, 133–134,
      141, 143–144
   in military, 143–144
   protection against, for research
      subjects, 133
Dishwashing, 166
Disinfection, 161, 165–166
DNA, 62, 63
Doctors. *See* Health care personnel
Drugs
   development and testing, 5,
      103–106
   intravenous. *See* Intravenous
      drug abusers
   new, 111–113
   previously developed, 106–111

Ear piercing, 100, 167
EBV (Epstein-Barr virus), 54, 83
Economic impact, 3–4, 7–8, 23,
   134–139
Eczema. *See* Weeping dermatitis
Education, for children with
   AIDS, 99–100, 122, 178–184
Educational programs
   on AIDS in children, 183–184
   funding for, 136–137
   for general population, 99–
      103, 117, 127–128
   for hemophiliacs, 94–95
   for high-risk groups, 91–95,
      126, 173
   for homosexuals, 91–93
   importance of starting, 117
   for individuals infected with
      HTLV-III/LAV, 98, 173–
      175
   for information on, 185–188
   for intravenous drug abusers,
      93–94, 174, 175
   for personal-service workers,
      167

Educational programs (*cont*)
   prevention by, 6–7, 90–91
   Red Cross, 9, 186
   responsibility for, 8–9, 136–
      137, 144–145
ELISA (enzyme-linked immuno-
   sorbent assay), 33–38, 149n,
   151n, 176
Emergency medical technicians,
   161–162. *See also* Health care
   personnel
Employment issues, 99, 168–169
Encephalitis, 44, 47
Encephalopathy. *See* Brain dis-
   ease
Envelope protein, 68–69, 114
Enzyme-linked immunosorbent
   assay (ELISA), 33–38, 176
Epidemic, development of, 12–
   19
Epstein-Barr virus (EBV), 54, 83
Equine infectious anemia virus,
   72
Esophagitis, 44, 150
Essex, Myron, 62, 115
Ethical issues, 144–145
Europe, incidence in, 16
Eviction, 121
Exudative lesions, 164, 167
Eye examinations, 100–101
Eye protection, 160

Factories, AIDS in, 99, 168
Families, transmission in, 10
Fauci, Anthony S., 58, 76, 84,
   85, 88, 117
Fear, 120, 123, 129–130
Fetus, transmission to, 11, 12,
   30, 180
Financial burdens, 3–4, 7–8, 23,
   134–139
Firefighters, 162
Folks, Thomas, 83
Food handling, 10, 155, 168, 182

Foscarnet, 109
Foster care, 178–184
Frazier, Shervert, 131
Funding, 7–8, 135–138
Fungal infections, 43, 150–151

Gallo, Robert C., 21, 58, 61–62, 63–65, 71, 73, 85, 88
Gamma interferon, 111
Garbage disposal, 161, 166
Geographic distribution, 2, 130–131, 163
Germicides, 165–166
Glial cells, 86
Gloves
  with children, 182
  for cleaning and waste disposal, 161, 166
  for health care workers, 160, 164
Goedert, James J., 2, 60
Gonorrhea, 24, 28, 90
Government policy. See Public health policy
Gowns, 160
Groopman, Jerome E., 117

Hairdressers, 100, 167
Haitians
  incidence in, 13, 18–19, 28, 39
  toxoplasmosis in, 45
Handshake, 10
Hardy, Ann M., 134
Haseltine, William, 69
Health care personnel
  fears of, 128–129
  infected, counseling of, 164–165
  precautions for, 100, 160–162, 164
  risk for, 31–32, 37, 159–160
  serologic testing of, 164
  stress on, 128–129
  transmission by, 163–165

Health care personnel (cont)
  transmission to, 10, 11, 31, 159–163
Health insurance, 138–139, 144
Heckler, Margaret M., 5–6
Helminthic infections, 150
Helper T cells. See T4 cells
Hemophiliacs
  educational programs for, 94–95
  as high-risk group, 26–27
  incidence in, 3, 13, 15, 26–27
  transmission by, 27
  transmission to, 26
Hepatitis B, 19, 61, 156, 157–159
Herpes simplex infection
  in children, 154
  in definition of AIDS, 44, 151
  in homosexuals, 45
Heterosexuals
  incidence in, 3, 17, 18
  partners of high-risk individuals, 27, 28
  promiscuity in, 12, 28–29
  transmission in, 11–12, 17, 27–29, 39
High-risk groups
  as blood donors, 12, 32
  children in, 29–30, 38–39, 56, 180–181
  counseling for, 95–97, 173–175
  defined, 23–30, 95–96, 156, 173
  educational programs for, 91–95, 173
  hemophiliacs as, 26–27
  homosexual men as, 23–25, 96–97
  infected individuals not in, 27–29
  intravenous drug abusers as, 25–26
  life expectancies in, 15
  partners of individuals in, 27, 28, 37

High-risk groups (*cont*)
  promiscuity in, 174
  prostitutes as, 18
  psychosocial effects on, 124–127
  reduction of transmission in, 173–176
  voluntary testing of, 95–97, 140, 173–174
Hirsch, Martin S., 117
Hispanics, incidence in, 14
Histiocytic tissue, cancer of, 154
Histoplasmosis, 151
Hodgkin's disease, 152, 154
Holland, Jimmie, 124
Home nursing care, 139, 161
Homosexual men
  as blood donors, 32
  changes in sexual behavior of, 24–25, 90–91, 124–125, 130
  discrimination against, 121–122, 133–134, 141, 143–144
  educational programs for, 91–93
  herpes infections in, 45, 54
  as high-risk group, 23–25, 96–97
  incidence in, 3, 24
  Kaposi's sarcoma in, 50
  screening test for, 96
  transmission in, 25, 60
Homosexual women, 30
Hospices, 139
Hospital care
  cost of, 23, 134, 138–139
  organization of, 138–139
Hotlines, 185–188
House arrest, 140, 142
Housing, 121, 122
HPA-23, 109–110
HTLV, 65, 67
HTLV-I, 65–66, 70, 71
HTLV-II, 65, 66, 70, 71
HTLV-III/LAV, 67n
  activation of, 84, 87–88

HTLV-III/LAV (*cont*)
  acute infection with, 51, 84
  antibody test for, 20–21, 33–38
  brain infection by, 22, 54–56, 85–87, 88
  comparison with hepatitis B virus, 157–159
  course of infection by, 83–85
  in definition of AIDS, 44–45
  disruption of immune function by, 78–85, 87
  diversity of, 68–69, 114
  education and foster care of children with, 178–184
  guidelines for infected individuals, 37, 84–85, 97
  identification of individuals with, 172–177
  immune response to, 85, 88, 114–115
  incidence of, 23
  isolation of, 65–68
  and lentiviruses, 70–72
  life cycle of, 73, 111
  lymphomas and, 53–54
  marker for, 105
  progression to ARC and AIDS, 21–22
  replication of, 69–70
Human T-cell leukemia/lymphoma virus (HTLV), 65. *See also* HTLV-I; HTLV-II
Human T-cell lymphotropic virus (HTLV), 67. *See also* HTLV-I; HTLV-II; HTLV-III/LAV
Humoral immune response, 75–76
Hypodermic needles. *See* Needles
Hypogammaglobulinemia, 154

Immune response
  cell-mediated, 75, 78, 79
  disruption by HTLV-III/LAV, 78–85, 87

Immune response (*cont*)
to HTLV-III/LAV, 85, 88,
114–115
humoral, 75–78
Immune stimulators, 110–111
Immune system
effects of AIDS on, 78–85, 87
healthy, 74–78
stress and, 7, 130
Immunity. *See* Immune response; Immune system
Immunization. *See* Vaccines
Immunodeficiency, causes of,
153–154
Immunofluorescent assay, 149n,
151n, 176
Immunosuppression, 110, 153–
154
Incidence of AIDS
in Africa, 16–18, 39
from blood transfusions, 3, 13,
32, 38–39
in children, 29
in Europe, 16
geographic, 2, 130–131, 163
in Haiti, 13, 18–19, 28
in hemophiliacs, 3, 13, 15, 26–
27
in heterosexuals, 3, 17, 18
in high-risk groups, 1–3, 13
in homosexual men, 3, 24
of HTLV-III/LAV, 23
after infection with HTLV-III/
LAV, 21–22
information on, 186
in intravenous drug abusers, 3,
15, 25
of unexplained cases, 27–29
in United States, 12, 14–15,
130–131
Incubation period
and acute infection with
HTLV-III/LAV, 51, 84
length of, 39, 57, 86
and public health policy, 39,
133
transmission during, 57

Infants
blood transfusions in, 38
diagnosis in, 56, 57
at risk, 56, 180
transmission to, 30, 180
vaccine intolerance in, 57
Information sources, 185–188.
See also Educational programs
Informed consent, 123
Insurance coverage, 138–139, 144
Intercourse
anal, 11, 60
vaginal, 11, 37
Interferons, 49, 107–109, 111
Interleukin-1, 77
Interleukin-2, 79, 111
Interstitial pneumonitis, chronic
lymphoid, 152
Intestinal inflammation, 44
Intravenous drug abusers
cases attributed to, 89
educational programs for, 93–
94, 174, 175
as high-risk group, 25–26
incidence in, 3, 15, 25
partners of, 27
transmission in, 25, 61, 93–94,
172–176
Invasive procedures, precautions
for, 163–164
Isoprinosine, 111
Isosporiasis, 152

Jaffe, Harold, 21
Job loss, 121
Johnson, Richard T., 58, 73, 88,
117

Kaposi's sarcoma
in Africa, 16–17, 50
in brain, 49
CMV infection and, 46, 50
in definition of AIDS, 44, 151,
154

Kaposi's sarcoma (*cont*)
  in homosexual men, 50
  incidence of, 49, 50–51, 54
  nitrite inhalants in, 97
  signs of, 49
  survival with, 49
  susceptibility to, 50
  treatment of, 49–50, 107
Kissing, 37, 102–103

Laboratory technologists. *See* Health care personnel
Lane, Clifford, 81, 82
Latency period. *See* Incubation period
Laundry, cleaning of, 166
Laundry workers. *See* Health care personnel
LAV (lymphadenopathy-associated virus), 66. *See also* HTLV-III/LAV
Law enforcement personnel, 161–162
Lee, Philip R., 146
Legal counseling, 122, 186
Legal issues, 8, 139–145, 180
Lentiviruses, 63, 70–72
Lesions, exudative, 164, 167
Leukemia
  lymphocytic, 154
  T-cell, 65–66
Leukoencephalopathy, progressive multifocal, 151
Levy, Jay, 67
Life expectancies, for high-risk groups, 15
Lifeguards, 162
Life-style, 60–61
Linens, cleaning of, 166
Lymphadenopathy, angioimmunoblastic, 154
Lymphadenopathy-associated virus (LAV), 66. *See also* HTLV-III/LAV

Lymphadenopathy syndrome, 51–53, 58
Lymphocyte transfers, 110
Lymphocytes, 75. *See also* B lymphocytes; T lymphocytes
Lymphocytic leukemia, 154
Lymphoid interstitial pneumonitis, chronic, 152
Lymphomas, 53–54, 58, 151, 152, 154
Lymphoreticular tissue, cancer of, 154

Macaques, STLV-III in, 115
Malnutrition, 154
Manicurists, 167
Masks, 160
Massage therapists, 167
McKusick, Leon, 91
Medical care
  cost of, 23, 134, 138–139
  organization of, 138–139
Medical examiners. *See* Health care personnel
Medical insurance, 138–139, 144
Memory loss, 54–56, 71, 86, 123
Men, incidence in, 14. *See also* Homosexual men
Meningitis, 44, 45, 56
Military, screening tests for, 140, 142–144
Monkeys
  STLV-III in, 72, 115–116
  transmission from, 72
Monocytes
  in AIDS, 80, 81–82, 87
  in normal immune response, 76–78, 79
Montagnier, Luc, 58, 66, 73, 88
Mops, 183
Moral issues, 144–145
Mortality rate, 2, 14, 42
Morticians. *See* Health care personnel

Mouth-to-mouth resuscitation, 100, 160, 162
Mucous membrane exposure, 159, 162–163, 164
Multifocal progressive leukoencephalopathy, 151
Multiple myeloma, 154
Mutation, in AIDS virus, 68–69, 114
Mycobactericidal disinfectant, 165–166
Mycobacterium avium-intracellulare, 47–48; 110, 151
Mycobacterium kansasii, 151
Myeloma, multiple, 154

Natural killer cells, 78, 80
Needles
    sharing of, 25, 61, 93–94
    sterilization of, 37, 93–94
Needle sticks
    and hepatitis B virus, 158
    and HTLV-III/LAV, 31, 159
    management of, 162–163, 164
    precautions to avoid, 160, 161
Neonates
    diagnosis in, 154
    transmission to, 11, 12, 30, 180
Nitrite inhalants, 60, 97
Non-Hodgkin's lymphoma, 54, 152
Nurses. *See* Health care personnel

Offices, AIDS in, 99, 168
Oncoviruses, 62–63, 71
Opportunistic infections
    with *Candida albicans,* 47
    in children, 181
    with cryptococcal meningitis, 45
    with *Cryptosporidium,* 48

Opportunistic infections (*cont*)
    with cytomegalovirus, 46–47
    defined, 42
    in definition of AIDS, 44, 149, 150–152
    descriptions of common, 45–48
    examples of, 41–42
    in HTLV-III/LAV-infected health care workers, 164–165
    with herpes infections, 45
    microorganisms causing, 43
    with *Mycobacterium avium-intracellulare,* 47–48
    pattern of, 42
    with *Pneumocystis carinii* pneumonia, 44, 45–46
    in T-cell leukemia, 66
    with toxoplasmosis, 45, 47
    with tuberculosis, 45, 48
Optometrists. *See* Health care personnel
Oral/genital contact, 11, 37
Organ donors, 12
Organizations, to contact for AIDS information, 185–188
Osborn, June E., 3, 4, 117, 126, 146

Pape, Jean, 18
Paralysis, 54, 86
Paramedics, 161–162. *See also* Health care personnel
Parasites, opportunistic infection by, 43
Parenteral exposure, 159, 162–163, 164
Pedicurists, 167
Personality changes, 123
Personal-service workers, 166–167
Phagocytes, 75, 76

Phagocytosis, 75
Phlebotomists. *See* Health care
    personnel
Physical limitations, 122–123
Physicians. *See* Health care per-
    sonnel
Pneumocystis carinii pneumonia,
    44, 45–46, 59, 150
Pneumonitis, chronic lymphoid
    interstitial, 152
Podiatrists. *See* Health care per-
    sonnel
Policy. *See* Public health policy
Popovic, Mikulas, 66
Pregnancy
    in health care workers, 160–
        161
    in high-risk individuals, 175
    in intravenous drug abusers,
        94
    in spouses of hemophiliacs, 95
Prevention
    by educational programs, 6–7,
        90–95, 99–103
    government's role in, 98–99,
        136
    after infection by HTLV-III/
        LAV, 84–85, 97
    by vaccine, 113–116
    by voluntary testing and coun-
        seling, 95–97, 140, 173–
        174
    in workplace, summary of
        PHS guidelines for, 155–
        156
Productivity loss, 3–4
Progressive multifocal leukoen-
    cephalopathy, 151
Promiscuity
    in Africa, 17, 18
    in heterosexuals, 12, 28–29
    in high-risk individuals, 174
    in homosexuals, 24–25, 90–91
    in military, 28–29
    and other infections, 19

Prostitutes
    as high-risk group, 18
    house arrest of, 140, 142
    intravenous drug abuse
        among, 25–26
    transmission by, 17, 28
Prostitution, houses of, 98, 176
Protozoal infections, 150
Psychosocial effects
    for AIDS patients, 119–123
    for ARC patients, 123–124
    examples of, 118–119
    for general population, 127–
        128
    for health care personnel, 128–
        129
    for high-risk individuals, 124–
        127
Public health policy
    on community versus individ-
        ual civil rights, 8, 139–
        145, 180
    on contact tracing, 8, 98–99,
        176
    coordination of, 137–138
    on costs and funding, 7–8, 23,
        134–139
    on educational materials, 8–9,
        136–137
    examples of issues in, 145
    options in, 140
    problems in developing, 132–
        134
    public attitude toward, 127–
        128, 134
    on regulation of high-risk es-
        tablishments, 97–98, 140–
        141, 176
    and social mores, 144–145
    on voluntary versus manda-
        tory measures, 8, 98–99,
        140
Public information programs.
    See Educational programs;
    Public health policy

Puncture wounds
  incidence of, 31
  management of, 162–163, 164

Quarantine, 8, 98, 140, 141–142

Radiation therapy, for Kaposi's
    sarcoma, 49
Razors, 37, 167, 175
Red Cross, 9, 186
Redfield, Robert, 28–29
Replication of HTLV-III/LAV,
    69–70
  drugs that inhibit, 107–110,
    111–113
Reporting, mandatory, 8, 125,
    175
Research
  on animal models, 115
  on brain infection, 85–87
  on existing drugs, 106–111
  funding for, 136, 137
  on HTLV-III/LAV virus, 65–
    73
  on immune function, 78–85
  on immune stimulators, 110–
    111
  on immunosuppressants, 110
  on new drugs, 111–113
  on susceptibility, 4
  on treatment, 103–113
  on vaccine, 113–116
Retroviruses, 61–65. See also
    Lentiviruses, Oncoviruses
Reverse transcriptase, 107, 108,
    109, 110, 112
Ribavirin, 109
Risk, after infection with HTLV-
    III/LAV, 21–22
Risk factors. See also High-risk
    groups
  for blood transfusions, 32–39
  for children, 29–30

Risk factors (cont)
  for health care workers, 31–32,
    37, 159–160
  for hemophiliacs, 26–27
  for homosexual men, 23–25
  for homosexual women, 30
  for intravenous drug abusers,
    25–26
  for partners of high-risk indi-
    viduals, 27
  promiscuity as, 12, 24–25, 28–
    29, 124
Risk-reduction education. See
    Educational programs
RNA, 62, 63
Rous, Francis Peyton, 62

Saliva, 11, 37, 102–103, 162
Sarcoma, 152. See also Kaposi's
    sarcoma
Schools, AIDS in, 99–100, 122,
    168, 178–184
Scott, Gwendolyn, 30
Screening tests. See also Testing
  for all patients, 163
  for blood donors, 12, 32–38
  for health care workers, 164
  for high-risk individuals, 95–
    97
  for military, 140, 142–144
Semen
  immunosuppression by, 60
  transmission in, 156
Servicemen, testing of, 140, 142–
    144
Service occupations, 166–168
Sex clubs, 140
Sexual behavior. See also Promis-
    cuity
  anal intercourse, 11, 60
  cases attributed to, 89
  changes in, 90–91, 93, 124–
    125, 130

Sexual behavior *(cont)*
  high-risk, 90
  oral/genital contact, 11, 37
  and T lymphocytes, 60
  and transmission, 6
  vaginal intercourse, 11, 37
Sexual partners, 27, 28, 37
Shooting galleries, 98, 176
Siblings, 10
Silverman, Mervyn F., 92, 117,
    140–141, 146
Simian T-lymphotropic virus
    type I (STLV-I), 65, 71–72
Simian T-lymphotropic virus
    type III (STLV-III), 71–72,
    115–116
Slim disease, 17
Sneezing, 10
Social effects. *See* Psychosocial
    effects
Sodium hypochlorite, 161, 166,
    168
Sperm donors, 12
Starvation, 154
Sterilization, of instruments
  for acupuncture needles, 37
  for dental instruments, 31–32
  in health care facilities, 165–
    166
  for hypodermic needles, 37,
    93–94
  in laboratories, 165–166
  for personal-service workers,
    167
STLV-I (simian T-lymphotropic
    virus type I), 65, 71–72
STLV-III (simian T-lymphotro-
    pic virus type III), 71–72,
    115–116
Stress
  for AIDS patients, 119–123
  for ARC patients, 123–124
  for general population, 127–
    128
  for health care personnel, 128–
    129

Stress *(cont)*
  for high-risk individuals, 124–
    127
  and immune function, 7, 130
Strongyloidosis, 150
Sulfa drugs, adverse reactions to,
    46
Support services, 122, 138–139,
    185–188
Suppressor cells, 78
Suramin, 107
Survival rate, 42
Susceptibility, 4, 130
Swollen glands, 51–53
Symptoms
  of AIDS, 44–45, 78, 149–154
  of AIDS-related complex
    (ARC), 19, 52
Syphilis, 28
Syringes. *See* Needles

tat-III gene, 70
Tattooing, 100, 167
T-cell leukemia, 65–66
Tears, transmission from, 11,
    156
Teenagers, educational programs
    for, 101–103
T8 cells, 78–81
Testing
  of all patients, 163
  with antibody tests, 20–21,
    33–38, 176
  for blood donors, 32–38
  confidentiality of, 125–126
  of food-service workers, 168
  of health care workers, 162,
    164
  of high-risk individuals, 95–
    97, 140, 173–174
  of infants, 57
  interpretation of, 176
  mandatory, 98, 140
  of partners, 37

Testing (*cont*)
of personal-service workers, 167
policy on reporting results of, 8
psychosocial impact of, 126–127
for school entrance, 183
of servicemen, 140, 142–144
sites for, 96
voluntary, 95–97, 140, 173–174
T4 cells
in AIDS, 60, 65, 78–81, 83–84, 87
function of, 76–78, 79
Thrush. *See* Candidiasis
Thymic hormones, 111
Tissues, disposable, 182–183
T lymphocytes
in AIDS, 60, 65, 66, 78–81, 83–85
cytotoxic, 75, 76, 78, 79, 85
function of, 75, 76–78, 79
Toothbrushes, 10, 37, 175
Towels, 182–183
Toxoplasmosis, 45, 47, 150, 154
trans-activator gene, 70
Transcriptase, reverse, 107, 108, 109, 110, 112
Transfusions. *See* Blood transfusions
Transmission
in blood, 65, 156
to blood donors, misconceptions about, 101
by casual contact, 10, 11, 156
to children, 11, 12, 29–30, 180–181
in day care, 181
by food-service workers, 168
in foster care, 181
to health care workers, 10, 11, 31, 159–163
from health care workers to patients, 163–165

Transmission (*cont*)
in hemophiliacs, 26
of hepatitis B virus, 157–159
in heterosexuals, 11–12, 17, 27–29, 39
in homosexual men, 25, 60
in intravenous drug abusers, 25, 61, 93–94, 172–176
modes of, 6, 10–12, 65
by personal-service workers, 166–167
reduction in high-risk groups, 173–176
from saliva, 11, 37, 102–103, 156
in schools, 181
in semen, 156
from tears, 11, 156
in workplace, 155–168
Treatment
by combination therapies, 111
difficulty in, 104–105, 106
with existing drugs, 106–111
by immune stimulators, 110–111
with new drugs, 111–113
outlook for, 5, 103
process of developing, 105–106
requirements for, 104, 117
Trisodium phosphonoformate, 109
Tross, Susan, 124
Tuberculosis, 45, 48

United States, incidence in, 12, 14–15, 130–131

Vaccines
and diversity of AIDS virus, 68–69
inability to tolerate, 57
research on, 113–116
risk of activating AIDS virus with, 84–85, 97, 183

Vaccines (*cont*)
  subunit, 113–114
  time frame for, 5–6, 116, 117
Viruses
  AIDS. *See* HTLV-III/LAV
  opportunistic infection by, 43,
    151
Visna viruses, 72, 86

Waiters, 155, 168
Waste disposal, 161, 165–166
Weeping dermatitis, 164, 167
Weiss, Stanley, 31

Western blot, 33, 35, 36, 149n,
  151n, 176
Whites, incidence in, 14
Women
  homosexual, 30
  incidence in, 14, 17, 18
  transmission by, 11, 17, 28–
    29, 39
  transmission to, 11–12, 39
Workplace, AIDS in, 99, 155–
  168

Yarchoan, Robert, 112